Occupational Therapy in the Treatment of Adult Hemiplegia

ORTRUD EGGERS
Occupational Therapist
Basel

Foreword: Dr. K. Bobath
Mrs. B. Bobath, M.B.E., T.C.S.P.

Illustrations: Brigitte Bessel, Reihen

Translation: Christine Diebel
Occupational Therapist
London

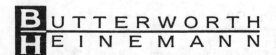

BUTTERWORTH
HEINEMANN

Butterworth-Heinemann Ltd
Linacre House, Jordan Hill, Oxford OX2 8DP

 PART OF REED INTERNATIONAL BOOKS

OXFORD LONDON BOSTON MUNICH
NEW DELHI SINGAPORE SYDNEY
TOKYO TORONTO WELLINGTON

First published 1983
Reprinted 1984, 1986, 1987, 1988, 1990, 1991

© Butterworth-Heinemann Ltd 1983

ISBN 0 7506 0128 0 ✓

Originally published by Springer-Verlag
(Berlin, Heidelberg, New York, Tokyo) as
Ergotherapie bei Hemiplegie, 2nd edition, 1982

Printed in Great Britain by Antony Rowe Ltd, Chippenham, Wiltshire

Contents

ACKNOWLEDGEMENTS

I should like to thank everyone who has helped me with this book.

Brigitte Bessel's clear illustrations complement the text and make it more understandable for the reader.

My special thanks go to Mrs Berta Bobath and her husband Dr. K. Bobath for the interest and encouragement they have shown towards applying their treatment concept in occupational therapy.

ORTRUD EGGERS

Foreword

The treatment of patients with upper motor neurone lesions, especially adults with hemiplegia, is a total programme, involving a variety of problems, such as activities of daily living, perception, speech and vocational training. It requires team-work and the close collaboration of physiotherapists, speech therapists and occupational therapists. For treatment to succeed all those who are concerned with a patient should follow the same basic concept and adopt the same principles of treatment.

The aim of treatment of the hemiplegic patient, as developed clearly in the introduction of this book, is not one of short term rehabilitation alone. This often neglects the hemiplegic side and is limited to giving the patient the possibility of self-help and independence by concentrating on compensatory activities of the non-affected side. There is, however, a large untapped potential on the affected side in most patients, which can be developed, even in long-standing cases of residual hemiplegia. This is done by inhibition of the abnormal patterns of spasticity and by facilitation and stimulation of normal automatic and voluntary functional movements. They are masked and interfered with by the patterns of spasticity and by sensory disturbances, the latter frequently associated with the motor handicap.

This book demonstrates in a clear and concise way, the value of involving an experienced occupational therapist, who is able to translate the work of the physiotherapist into functional and vocational activity, thus complementing physiotherapy. Moreover, the author shows the importance of assessing the sensory-perceptory deficits for gauging the results of treatment, prognosis and progress.

The book is well illustrated, with detailed explanations of the gradual development and build-up of manipulation in treatment. We have long awaited this book, which meets a need in the area of total management by relating physiotherapy and occupational therapy. It will be of special value to occupational therapists who are working in hospitals where each member of the team follows the same concept and principles. We wish the book every success.

Karel and Berti Bobath
The Bobath Centre, London.

Introduction

Of the numerous disabilities that are treated in occupational therapy, adult hemiplegia forms a relatively large group. As the average age of the population and injuries caused by road traffic accidents increase, more and more brain-damaged patients of all ages are referred to occupational therapy for rehabilitation.

The cause of a hemiplegia is always an injury to the central nervous system, but the resultant deficits vary from patient to patient. Several of these are treated, or at least taken into consideration, in occupational therapy, but only a small part of the vast topic is described in this book. It is the sensory-motor disability of these patients and their treatment in occupational therapy that are looked at in detail. In particular, the treatment of the arm and hand and its relation to the application of movement in all activities of daily living forms the basis of functional occupational therapy. Functional improvement of arm and hand can only be achieved, however, if head, neck, trunk, and legs – in fact the whole person – are incorporated into treatment. A detailed analysis of the disability is essential in order to establish correctly the individual treatment, aims and objectives.

Other published work is usually limited to one-handed activities of daily living (ADL) and work techniques, and if the occupational therapist wants to treat the sensory-motor deficits of a hemiplegic patient it is difficult to find information about how to do this. In order to fill this need, this book describes the treatment experiences using the Bobath concept that have been collected over a number of years.

It is impossible for colleges of occupational therapy to go into the detail of each specialised area. So much has to be learned that it is not surprising that qualified occupational therapists, on the whole, have little knowledge about specialised treatment of hemiplegia. A certain knowledge of neurophysiology, pathology and of normal movement is a prerequisite.

The treatment suggestions are not a 'fail-safe' recipe that can be applied to all hemiplegic patients, and it is necessary to adapt treatment to the specified deficits and the individual patient's needs. Short and long-term treatment aims of inpatients as well as outpatients also need to be considered by the therapist.

The illustrations always show a patient with a right-sided hemiplegia.

This book does not claim to be comprehensive, but through it therapists will gain a better understanding of the treatment of the specific problems of an adult hemiplegic patient. The theme is a very practical one.

I am certain that some of my colleagues have different or additional experiences in this field and I should be delighted to hear from them.

I The Role of Occupational Therapy in Rehabilitation

A. Links between occupational therapy and other professions
B. The doctor and occupational therapy
C. Nursing and occupational therapy
D. Physiotherapy and occupational therapy
E. Speech therapy and occupational therapy
F. Social work and occupational therapy
G. The psychologist and occupational therapy
H. Vocational guidance and occupational therapy
I. Relatives and occupational therapy
J. Harmony within the team
K. Team conferences

The medical, social and vocational rehabilitation of the brain-injured adult is the concern of all members of the rehabilitation team. The most important member of this team is the disabled person himself. With his (or her) specific physical disability, the hemiplegic patient is at the centre of all treatment procedures. The personality of the patient, his psychological and social circumstances are all taken into account.

The rehabilitation team may consist of the doctor, nurses, physiotherapist, occupational therapist, speech therapist, the social worker, psychologist and vocational guidance officer (or disabled resettlement officer — DRO). In addition, the relatives and friends of the patient play an important part in the long-term therapy.

According to the individual needs of the patient, not all the different modes of treatment may be required and the intensity of treatment may vary. Nevertheless, all these specialists are respected by each other as essential and equal members of the rehabilitation team. Everyone taking part in the treatment process has the same aim — the best possible rehabilitation of the hemiplegic patient. There is a difference, however, in that each discipline aims at this goal from a particular point of view. Hence, only if the individual experts can look at their function in relation to, and not in isolation from, one another can an integrated and common goal be reached.

Occupational therapists are a link in this chain of specialists. Little is generally known about our function, so it is our duty to inform our colleagues in the team of the contribution that the occupational therapist can make towards the rehabilitation of the hemiplegic patient.

A. Links Between Occupational Therapy and Other Professions

Today, with specialisation, there are clear demarcations among the professions. Even so, there are points of contact and overlap because fundamentally all are striving to reach the same treatment goals. A well-functioning rehabilitation team is one where the transition of the patient from one treatment mode to another is smooth.

B. The Doctor and Occupational Therapy

As leader and coordinator of all rehabilitation procedures, it is the duty of the doctor, firstly, to know which therapies are available and, secondly, to assess the optimum moment of referral of the patient to them.

Either from the doctor himself or through reading the medical notes, one should get detailed information about the patient's condition. This information should include such things as precautions, drugs and contraindications. As with all aspects of the patient's treatment — for example, results of laboratory tests — the doctor expects feedback. A report by the occupational therapist may be given direct to the doctor or within the team meeting.

C. Nursing and Occupational Therapy

Links with the nursing staff occur mostly during the positioning and 'activities of daily living' (ADL) training of the patient.

The occupational therapist can advise on both the most suitable sitting position for the patient in a chair and on the best position for his affected arm while he is on the ward, during treatment-free time.

In order that the hemiplegic patient may again learn to eat, wash and dress independently, the occupational therapist should work closely with the nursing staff so that correct procedures may be reinforced on the ward. This means a frequent exchange of information regarding the level of independence that the patient has reached and which aids are required to maintain this level.

Details about sensory disturbances that are discovered in occupational therapy should be conveyed to the nursing staff so that burns and other injuries may be avoided.

D. Physiotherapy and Occupational Therapy

Both forms of therapy follow basically the same treatment aim — that is, the improvement of motor function.

The physiotherapist encourages equally the basic movement of trunk, upper and lower extremities. The retraining of walking patterns with control of head, trunk and arm takes place in physiotherapy, as does the initial relearning of arm and hand movements.

The occupational therapist concerns herself with the practical application of these movements. This practical training includes not only physical control of head, trunk and lower extremity but the psychological, social and perceptual problems of each patient are also considered.

To achieve the best result for the patient, cooperation between therapists is most important. This means that the same treatment aim should be used by both disciplines, i.e. working for symmetry and function of the affected side rather than the compensatory training of the sound side while ignoring the affected side. Such contradictory therapy would clearly confuse the patient.

E. Speech Therapy and Occupational Therapy

The specific treatment of aphasia in a hemiplegic patient is carried out by the speech therapist. The occupational therapist may again give advice on both sitting and arm positions of a patient while in speech therapy. The speech therapist may give the occupational therapist and other team members instructions regarding the most suitable approach to take with severely speech-handicapped patients.

Impaired writing ability may be due either to the motor disability of the dominant hand, or to the disorder of aphasia, or it may be a combination of both. In severe cases there might also be additional disabilities caused by lack of form-perception and form-construction. After consultation between both therapists, the appropriate time can be chosen for writing training to begin. Usually it is in occupational therapy that the patient practises the movements needed for fluent writing. This may be done by using either the returning function of the affected limb, or the non-dominant hand. Improvement of the written content, however, is a part of the treatment of aphasia that belongs in the domain of speech therapy.

F. Social Work and Occupational Therapy

The social worker is responsible for the patient's affairs during the transition from medical rehabilitation to resettlement back into the community. The occupational therapist can help the social worker by communicating all relevant information regarding the patient. This would relate to his independence in all activities of daily living and mobility, as well as aids and adaptations that will be needed either at home or at work.

G. The Psychologist and Occupational Therapy

The neuropsychologist can test psychological brain function by using a standardised test. The results of this test — in addition to her own observations of the patient — are valuable for planning treatment by the occupational therapist. Details of performance relating to memory, concentration, learning ability, sequencing, ability to adapt, and spatial thinking, allow the occupational therapist to achieve the optimum working level without putting excessive demands on the patient.

The training of specific brain function is usually done by occupational therapists, although in some hospitals this may be done by the psychologist. In either case, the occupational therapist will be concerned with the practical improvement of these functions and many areas in occupational therapy can be used for this. Three-dimensional constructional ability may, for example, be tested in woodwork, and memory can be tested by asking a patient to follow a recipe by reading each instruction once.

In addition to the above, cooperation between the occupational therapist, the psychologist and, in some cases, the psychiatrist, is extremely valuable when dealing with the psychological problems of the patient.

H. Vocational Guidance and Occupational Therapy

Vocational guidance is necessary when a patient is unable to return to his former occupation, or if, as a result of his disability, changes need to be made in order for him to return to it.

The occupational therapist should inform the DRO of any special qualifications, abilities and interests the patient may have, and also any limitations which have been observed in occupational therapy. The rehabilitation programme in occupational therapy should include improvement of skills necessary to return to the same kind of job, or the learning of new skills for alternative employment.

I. Relatives and Occupational Therapy

Occupational therapy should include the relatives, the more they are involved in treatment the more they will understand the nature of the disability. This will benefit the patient and the relatives by enabling the treatment aims to be carried on after discharge.

J. Harmony Within the Team

The cooperation, motivation and insight of the patient are vital if the optimum rehabilitation goal is to be reached. How then can treatment promote this? The active participation by the individual in his treatment is best achieved if he is convinced that all the disciplines concerned have the same short-term and long-term goals. The instructions and explanations which the patient receives from doctors, nurses, and therapists, should therefore be the same.

The first impression that the patient gets when referred to the various therapists is very important. It is crucial that the doctor presents and explains clearly the value of the different rehabilitative measures.

An Example of a Bad Referral to Occupational Therapy would be: 'So Mrs M., from now on you will attend occupational therapy daily for one hour. There you can make nice things, so that you will not become bored. While this side of yours is paralysed you will work with your good hand. The occupational therapist will also show you how you can get dressed (and undressed) one-handed!'

If the patient is sitting completely asymmetrically in his wheelchair when occupational therapy begins, it is not possible to start the training of activities of daily living due to a lack of sitting balance. The occupational therapist chooses bilateral activities to enlarge the patient's movement radius and improve sitting balance. This is a preparation for undressing and dressing, as well as functional training of the paralysed arm. One would therefore expect the patient to be disappointed with this sort of occupational therapy because the expectations given by the doctor are not met. This may cause frustration and therefore a lack of cooperation.

There is an Alternative Example: 'So Mrs M., as you are now able to sit out of bed for a few hours each day I would like you to have occupational therapy as well as physiotherapy. You will work mainly with your paralysed arm and hand, but in the beginning your sound hand will have to help and therefore you will work with both hands. The occupational therapist will show you how you can use your paralysed side during activities. As soon as your sitting balance has improved and you can safely bend forward, the occupational therapist will show you how to dress and undress including, for example, how to fasten your shoelaces with one hand.'

Through good communication, realistic goals must be established by the rehabilitation team. All measures should be sensibly considered — for example, an aphasic patient should not be referred to occupational therapy for one-handed typewriting training if the speech therapist thinks that his understanding of reading and writing is insufficient. Another example would be if a nurse and a physiotherapist think that a patient should be able to dress himself independently but the occupational therapist considers that this is impossible because the patient has gross body scheme problems. Excessive demands and unsuitable treatment will lead to frustration and disappointment for the patient and result in lack of motivation. It is vital that the different specialists establish a well-balanced and well-adjusted treatment plan for each individual patient.

The Bobath treatment method is a most productive one if all the team members use it as far as it is applicable in their line of work. The transfer of the patient from bed to wheelchair, for example, should always be carried out in exactly the same way by physiotherapist, occupational therapist and nurses, as well as by relatives. Otherwise the patient may be instructed by one therapist to use and take weight on the affected side, while another therapist allows him to ignore the affected side completely. It is essential that each team member knows the treatment aims and methods of the other disciplines and has confidence in his own as well as those of his colleagues.

K. Team Conferences

The intensity of, and the methods used by, each individual therapy must be adapted to the degree of the disability as well as the psychological and physical ability of the patient. For example, a patient has, in line with his disability, the following therapy programme: physiotherapy twice a day; ADL training a.m.; remedial occupational therapy p.m.; speech therapy once or twice a day. The therapist has to judge whether this kind of programme is reasonable or too demanding. If it is thought to be unreasonable, the whole team should discuss which therapies are most important at that particular stage of treatment and the programme should be altered accordingly. Progress and regression should also be discussed at these meetings.

II Treatment Using Bobath Principles

There are different ways of treating an adult hemiplegic patient. Each method has its own specific treatment principles, which are developed in accordance with the way in which the founder saw the problems and which ones they emphasised.

The Bobath concept has impressed me and I am so convinced of its effectiveness in the treatment of hemiplegic patients that I have made it the basis of treatment for the last 12 years, as well as the basis of this book.

It is impossible to describe the Bobath principles in detail here, but a book* describing them is widely available. For the reader who is totally unfamiliar with this treatment technique, a brief description follows: Dr Bobath, a neurologist, and his wife, a physiotherapist, developed their treatment concept for cerebral palsied children and adult hemiplegia after the Second World War and today it is recognised worldwide. Although the treatment for children differs from the treatment of an adult, the principles are basically the same. The aim is not the compensatory training of the sound side but the facilitation of movement on the hemiplegic side, trying to achieve symmetry of body and movement. With this method, abnormal posture and movement patterns are inhibited and therefore spasticity is reduced and normal movement sequences may be facilitated. These are at first carried out with the guidance of the therapist and, through repetition, once more become automatic.

The patient knows only abnormal postures and movements and can only carry them out with different degrees of spasticity. With these patterns, normal movement is impossible: therefore it is crucial to inhibit spasticity before facilitation of normal movement can begin. It

* Berta Bobath, (1980). *Adult Hemiplegia: Evaluation and Treatment*. London: William Heinemann Medical Books.

is important for the patient that during treatment he regains a feeling for normal muscle tone and normal posture, as well as normal movement; through this he gets normal sensory-motor experiences. To achieve this the therapist chooses reflex inhibiting postures and movements. At the beginning the therapist guides the movements of the patient through manipulation techniques, thereby preventing any recurrence of the abnormal pattern until the patient is able to control this himself. The whole body should be taken into consideration during treatment. The therapist always inhibits proximally to distally — for example, one begins with the head then trunk, shoulder and hip. This is important because therapy can influence and reduce spasticity distally through proximal inhibition. These reflex inhibiting positions are not static but are starting positions for normal movements.

Sensory deficits are taken into consideration in the Bobath concept, as the sensory feedback between central nervous system and periphery is all-important.

Treatment cannot be standardised as each patient is an individual and has his own specific disability. The establishment of an individual treatment plan is based on detailed assessment and observation, feeling and correction of abnormal patterns and the facilitation of normal movement. The Bobath concept is not a fixed method but a technique that tries to overcome the difficulties of each individual adult hemiplegic patient.

This concept, which was developed for physiotherapists, can, in my opinion, be well incorporated into occupational therapy because it has the facilitation of normal movement sequences, which are necessary for all activities of daily living, as the goal. It can also improve cooperation between all the therapists and nursing staff, provided that all team members use this concept as a baseline.

III The Motor Problems of Hemiplegia and their Treatment

A. Motor problems
B. Treatment
C. Comparison of various motor problems and their treatment

A. Motor Problems

All occupational therapists working with adult hemiplegic patients know, more or less, the typical postures and movement patterns that result from this condition. Even so, I should like to go into the motor problems in depth in order to arrive at a common basis for suitable treatment aims and suggestions.

Changed motor function is due to partial loss of cortical control. This manifests itself with different pathological symptoms, and these differ greatly. Not every stroke patient has all the typical motor problems, and the various deficits have a negative effect on each other and cause new additional problems. Lack of movement often accompanies sensory deficits. Despite the difference in the degree of disability, most hemiplegic patients show similar features with regard to posture and motor problems and this makes the execution of normal movement difficult.

The typical abnormal characteristics will be broken down individually later on. This will help in the understanding of the complex nature of the disability. During treatment the total combined effect of the individual problems should be taken into consideration and the patient should be treated as a whole.

The occupational therapist should observe in the hemiplegic patient how his posture and movements differ from those of a healthy person. It is also important to promote the residual sound movements as well as to recognise abnormal posture and movements and, through treatment, to improve them.

B. Treatment

Traditionally, the treatment of an adult hemiplegic patient in physiotherapy and occupational therapy consisted mainly of compensatory training. The patient was taught to compensate with the sound side for loss of function on the affected side.
Examples
   During early walking with a stick, weight was only carried on the sound side.
   In early occupational therapy only one-handed training was carried out.
   By ignoring the hemiplegic side the abnormal posture of the hemiplegic patient became even more pronounced. With that kind of treatment the progress in the rehabilitation of the hemiplegic ended rapidly.

That approach is in direct contrast with the method used today. In order to have a symmetrical human being the emphasis is on inhibiting the abnormal postural reactions and facilitating more normal ones.

C. Comparison of Various Motor Problems and their Treatment

Suggestions for appropriate treatment of these problems can be found under 1 – 7b. Only by recognising the motor problems does one have the opportunity to influence them therapeutically.

Motor Problems	*Treatment*
(1a) Neglect of the hemiplegic side	(1b) Orientation towards the hemiplegic side
(2a) Asymmetry: lack of balance	(2b) Symmetry: training for balance
(3a) Abnormal movement	(3b) Facilitation of normal movement
(4a) Mass movements	(4b) Selective arm and hand function

(5a) Missing automatic reactions	(5b) Facilitation of automatic reactions
(6a) Lack of coordination in both hands	(6b) Useful coordination of both hands
(7a) Sensory deficits	(7b) Facilitation of tactile– kinaesthetic perception

(1a) Neglect of the Hemiplegic Side

After a stroke the hemiplegic patient is suddenly confronted with two halves of his body, which he perceives differently and which no longer work together. From the affected side, wrong or no information reaches the cortex and therefore impulses cannot be sent to the periphery. The two halves of the body are out of harmony but at the same time may influence each other negatively.

The patient feels insecure and tends to orientate himself towards the sound side. If there is also a sensory deficit the affected side is totally neglected. (Motor and sensory functions are closely linked, more detail is given under 7a in this Chapter.) Sensation in one side of the body does not correspond with sensation in the other and therefore the interplay between the two halves is lost. The patient's awareness of his affected side is drastically reduced and he becomes afraid of falling because he cannot rely on previously learned experiences. Some patients overestimate their abilities and fall because they are over-confident.

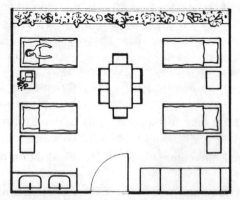

Figure 1. *Suitable position of the bed for a patient with right sided hemiplegia.*

Examples. Equilibrium reactions are present on the sound side whereas there are none on the affected side.

Because of passivity of the disabled side, more activity is demanded of the sound side and this results in an increased spasticity on the affected side through associated reactions (more details under 3a).

Activity is the focal point of occupational therapy and is an important component of daily life. Uncontrolled activity will reinforce the disability of these patients. Using the sound side and neglecting the hemiplegic side will encourage abnormal movements rather than inhibit them. The existence of the two halves working against instead of with each other presents special problems for the hemiplegic patient, and neglect of the affected side is a more or less common factor with all patients suffering from this disability.

(1b) Orientation Towards the Hemiplegic Side

To make the patient aware of his neglected side all stimuli should be directed towards it. The stimuli may be visual, auditory or tactile–kinaesthetic. The first step is the right choice of positioning of the bed on the ward.

By adapting the environment of the patient, most of the stimuli from it will come to him via the affected side. There is his personal locker, which he turns to frequently. Conversation with fellow patients, medical staff and visitors should occur on the affected side and they should always approach him from that side. All normal activity on the ward offers stimuli which make it possible for the hemiplegic patient to orientate himself towards the affected side (Fig 1).

Positioning. Positioning of the hemiplegic arm is important, not only during treatment sessions but also during the rest of the day. The arm should be positioned in the visual field of the patient so that it can be visually controlled. When the patient sits at the table the paralysed arm should never be *under* the table but *on* it. The correct positioning of the arm is always done by the patient himself and not by anyone else. Through this kind of positioning the affected side is encouraged back into awareness. The arm should always be positioned, including during speech therapy and while eating on the ward.

Bilateral Activities. It is often the patient with a complete spastic or flaccid lesion who shows obvious neglect of the hemiplegic side with no controlled function on the affected side. At this stage of the disability, bilateral activities with clasped or flat hands are particularly suitable.

During early treatment attention should be drawn to the hemiplegic side in order to achieve integration between the right and left halves of the body. Bilateral activities contribute towards this and make the patient more aware of his paralysed side. There is a good chance of recovery, especially if there is only minimal sensory loss.

In spite of this orientation towards the hemiplegic side, the therapist must obviously allow the sound hand to be used for self-help training and during other activities, but never without taking the affected side into consideration. The occupational therapist should advise the nursing staff that the patient should wash and dry himself even while still on bedrest. If a nurse helps with dressing she should ensure that the patient himself puts his affected arm into his sleeve with the help of his unaffected hand. These early activities again aim at making the patient more aware of his neglected side.

There is a danger of all activities such as rolling from supine into side-lying or prone, sitting up, standing and walking, being initiated with the automatic reactions of the sound side. Those reactions are missing on the affected side and *with this compensatory overactivity of the sound side no movement at all is initiated on the affected side*. An example of this is the movement from lying to sitting up, when the patient will support himself only with the sound arm and hand and not with the affected one, so that all the weight is on the sound side. *This overactivity on the sound side must be stopped in order to give the affected side the chance to become active*. To begin with, this is achieved by encouraging a balanced symmetrical distribution of weight in lying, sitting, standing and walking. At the same time, weight should be brought over the affected side so that automatic reactions like sitting up may be initiated. Only when this weight transfer is mastered to some extent in sitting, can function of the arm be prepared for through movement of trunk and shoulder girdle. Extension in the arm and hand is essential in order to make weightbearing on the arm possible and this can be practised during sitting and standing and during some remedial activities.

(2a) Asymmetry: Lack of Balance

As a result of the spastic lesion, asymmetry of body posture develops. Parts of the body that do not have normal sensation are not used normally.

During sitting, different forms of body asymmetry can arise: during the flaccid stage, most of the bodyweight falls towards the affected side; and during the spastic stage, pelvis and shoulder girdle approach each other due to flexor spasticity (Figs 2; 6a).

The result is similar if the patient passively uses his bodyweight to balance himself when there is lack of stability in trunk and hip. To prevent a fall towards the sound side while sitting, the trunk and head are bent towards the unaffected side. In the beginning the patients are more afraid of this than of falling onto the unaffected side. This asymmetrical posture very often results in back pain.

Due to lateral flexion of the head, the face is also turned towards the unaffected side. Because of this the patient loses visual control over the affected side and it therefore ceases to exist for him.

It is important, therefore, to remember that a hemiplegia is not just 'an arm and a leg' but head, neck and trunk are also involved. The whole of the affected side rotates backwards and the patient moves diagonally in space leading with the sound side, leaving the affected side behind. The abnormal posture of head, neck, shoulder girdle and pelvis have a negative effect on the functional ability of the extremities. Because of this asymmetry, body scheme and contact with the environment, including other people, are disturbed.

Although the analysis, as well as the treatment, of standing and walking belongs more to the area of physiotherapy, the occupational therapist should also know about it. When the patient is standing it is obvious that weight is only taken over the sound side. The result is increased extensor spasticity in the leg on the hemiplegic side resulting in loss of balance.

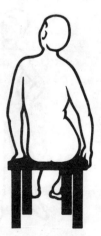

Figure 2. *Asymmetry of trunk, neck and head, with unequal weight distribution.*

During walking the therapist can distinguish between the 'stance phase' and the 'swing phase' of the leg. Extensor spasticity prevents adequate balance reactions if the hemiplegic leg is in the 'stance phase'. The resulting inadequate balance forces the patient to make a quick step with the sound leg because it is possible for him to bear weight on the affected side for only a very short time.

In the 'swing phase' the extended hemiplegic leg is brought forward by circumduction, because selection of flexion and extension movements is affected in the leg (Fig 3b). The 'hitching' of the hip, combined with the depression of the shoulder, results in shortening of the trunk on the same side. This results in an impairment of trunk-rotation which is needed during walking to retain balance. This rotation is also necessary for the natural 'swing' of the arm during walking.

The typical picture of asymmetry, lack of equilibrium reactions and unequal steps is reinforced when walking quickly or over uneven ground. Walking is described by Bobath as 'a constant losing and regaining of balance'.

The abnormal asymmetrical posture and movement patterns show clearly that it is not possible for a hemiplegic to have a normal equilibrium in sitting, standing and walking. The patient who is orientated during all his activities towards his sound side promotes the development of spastic patterns on the affected side and, unfortunately, at the same time this prevents the incorporation of normal postural and balance reactions.

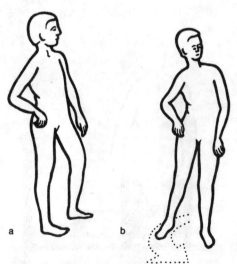

a   b

Figures 3a and 3b. *Asymmetry during stance and swing phase of the leg in walking.*

(2b) Symmetry: Training for Balance

Symmetry is promoted in the early stages if the affected side is incorporated — for example, through weight transfer and the training for balance movements.

Positioning in Bed. This is carried out by the nursing staff with the guidance of the physiotherapists.

The bed should be flat. A pillow under the neck prevents lateral flexion of the head toward the hemiplegic side. The back may be supported with a pillow. The affected shoulder should be brought forward, arm extended and laid down at right angles to the body. As a variation of the shoulder position, the fingers may be positioned under the pillow on which the sound leg is resting. The affected hip is extended and the knee is flexed.

Lying on the affected side has been proved to be useful for simple occupational therapy activities in bed (Fig 4).

Advantages
   Large movement radius of the sound arm
   Facilitation of sensation and proprioception through lying on the affected side
   Prevention of abnormal patterns and associated reactions

Correct Sitting Position. As soon as the patient is able to sit up for several hours a day, good positioning is vital in both chairs and wheelchairs, both on the ward and during treatment. All chairs should have a horizontal seat and backrest at a right angle (see Fig 5a).

The height and depth of the seat should be adjusted according to the height of the patient. If a patient has very short thighs, for example, the seat should be shortened with a hard backcushion; if the feet do not reach the ground a footstool or shortening of the footrest of the

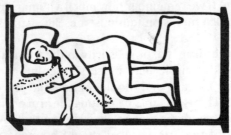

Figure 4. *Positioning in bed lying on the hemiplegic side.*

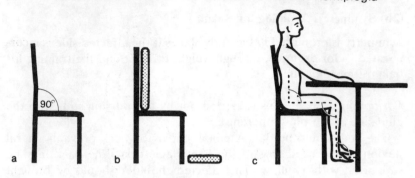

Figures 5a, 5b and 5c. *The adapted chair.*

wheelchair is necessary (Fig 5b). The patients have to learn to bend their hips sufficiently and not to extend their legs on the affected side. Hip, knee and ankle joints should all be at right angles to prevent extensor spasticity in the leg. The patient's bottom should be as far back as possible on the seat and it is also important that the patient sit in the middle of the seat and weight be equally distributed over both buttocks.

During treatment sessions the patient has to learn to get a feeling for symmetry, and has to be reminded to regain it if it is lost until he is able to control this himself. It is important to ensure symmetrical head, neck and trunk posture. There should not be a twisting of the body axis and especially no retraction of the scapula. The hemiplegic leg often falls into abduction and external rotation and this results in the inversion of the foot (Figs 6a, 6b).

Positioning of the Arm. The positioning of the arm on the table has already been mentioned in (1b). This is important for the awareness of the affected side. The correct positioning of the arm is particularly important in the early stages in order to achieve symmetrical body and shoulder posture. If we remember how much a human arm weighs then it is clear how much pull is on tendons, muscles, nerves and the joint capsule.

The weight of the arm, flexor spasticity in the trunk and the depression of the shoulder girdle may cause shortening of the trunk. To achieve symmetry in trunk and shoulder girdle the pull of the arm has to be eliminated. This is possible by putting the arm on a table (Fig 5c). If the patient sits mainly in a wheelchair during the day and if he has severe paralysis of the arm, a table should be made which is large enough to accommodate the whole forearm.

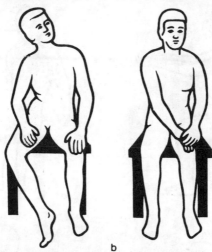

a   b

Figures 6a and 6b. *(a) Incorrect positioning of the leg through abduction and external rotation at the hip; the foot is inverted. (b) Correct positioning of the leg; the knee is in line with the toes.*

Change of Habits. There are certain routines which should be encouraged and observations that should be made — for example, the position of furniture in a room, and from which side the patient is approached on the ward and in occupational therapy. If incorrect, these factors will influence the symmetry of the patient.

Equilibrium in Sitting. The whole body is used actively to retain a good sitting posture. If equilibrium reactions are not present it is practised systematically in occupational therapy by weight transfers in all directions.

The first step is for the patient to learn not to use the backrest and to lean forward (Figs 7a; 13; 22; 23; 25; 32; 36; 72).

The next step, which is more difficult, is the weight transfer from right to left. It is often difficult for the patient to return from the diagonal to the vertical position (Fig 7c).

Rotation movements of the trunk are incorporated into the training of sitting balance (Fig 7d). These trunk rotations are extremely important for keeping equilibrium, and also have a positive influence on the movement functions of trunk and extremities. They are as follows.

Improvement of sitting balance;
Improvement of body awareness;
Preparation for standing and walking; and
Mobilisation of shoulder girdle.

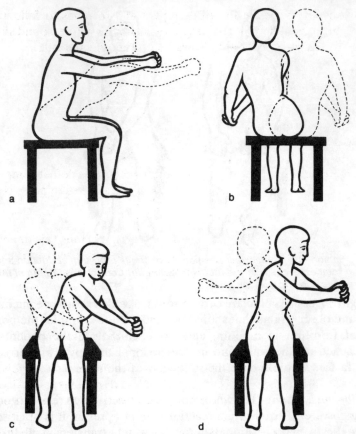

Figures 7a, 7b, 7c and 7d. *(a) Weight transfer in sitting, forwards and backwards. (b) Weight transfer in sitting to the side right and left. (c) Weight transfer in sitting with diagonal movements. (d) Weight transfer in sitting with trunk rotation.*

Through the correct choice of occupational therapy activities the therapist can systematically encourage sitting balance by, for example, block printing. Blocks and working surface are placed by the therapist so that the desired movements are encouraged (Fig 29). This demands a greater movement radius with appropriate posture changes of head, neck, trunk, arms and legs.

Good sitting balance is also the prerequisite for washing and dressing.

The training of walking patterns, which is different for each individual, is practised by physiotherapists. They may advise the occupational therapist how she can facilitate and control walking with each individual.

There is one principle for all therapists and relatives to follow: a hemiplegic patient does not need supporting on his active, sound side. If help is necessary it should always be on the affected side.

(3a) Abnormal Movement

Abnormal postural tone
Lack of coordination
Associated reactions

A lesion in the central nervous system often results in a deficit in motor control. The three effects mentioned above influence each other considerably.

Abnormal Postural Tone. Postural tone is the kind of tone that enables our muscles to hold certain positions as well as to adjust actively during changes in posture. This normal postural tone is necessary to regain equilibrium after each movement, even if it is only very slight. If a lesion of the central nervous system is present, this postural tone may be affected.

At the beginning, muscle tone is reduced and presents itself as a flaccid hemiplegia. Nevertheless, sooner or later most patients will have an increase in tone which, during passive movements, is felt as resistance and which makes active goal-directed movements difficult. Not all muscles, or only a single muscle, are affected by this hypertonus but it shows itself in a typical distribution over a whole muscle group. The abnormal muscle tone, whether flaccid or spastic, may affect the

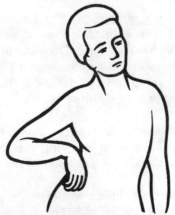

Figure 8. *Abnormal posture of the arm.*

whole side of the body. How spasticity affects head, trunk and the lower extremity was described under (2a).

In the arm the flexors are mainly affected, which results in the typical posture and movement patterns of a hemiplegic patient (Fig 8).

Shoulder Retraction. The scapula is pulled towards the spinal column. This can be observed frequently in most patients with spasticity and is often an explanation of why the affected arm glides off the table.

Shoulder Depression. Through spasticity in the trunk flexors the scapula is also pulled downwards. This makes trunk rotation and reaching beyond the midline difficult for the patient.

Internal Rotation and Adduction of the Shoulder. Patients sometimes show a combination of internal rotation with abduction.

Elbow flexion
Pronation
Wrist Flexion
Finger Flexion
Thumb Adduction

These are the typical movement patterns of a hemiplegic patient. As each individual is different, however, variations may occur.

Spasticity makes normal movements difficult or impossible and it also changes with each change of posture. It may vary in lying, sitting or standing and the psychological condition of the patient may influence it as well. It is therefore necessary for the therapist to establish which postures and movements increase, and which ones decrease, spasticity.

Lack of Coordination. For coordination of movements 'reciprocal innervation' is necessary. This is the fine-graded interplay between agonist and antagonist which makes normal movement possible. If the agonist is innervated the antagonist is usually inhibited. Through hypertonus in one muscle group and lack of tone in the antagonist the coordination between the two is disrupted.

Associated Reactions. These are stereotype reactions that reinforce the spastic pattern due to an increase in tone and may be the result of insecurity; effort; excitement; fear; overactivity of the sound hand; or pain.

The 'movements' that occur during associated reactions are the result of spasticity and should not be called movements but pathological reactions. Most patients find it difficult to understand that these associated reactions are undesirable and should be avoided.

Associated reactions should not be confused with normal associated movements. Examples of normal associated movements are movements of the tongue during writing; a mother may open her mouth while feeding her child; or the patient may open his sound hand when asked to release an object with the affected one.

These natural associated movements may stop voluntarily at any time. The abnormal associated reactions, however, cannot be influenced at will by the patient. As long as the patient is in the flaccid stage, these are not present. Only with the appearance of spasticity will associated reactions occur and first signs can be observed when a patient is coughing, sneezing or yawning.

Incorrect positioning, excessive demand on the patient during activity, anger or fear as well as isolated one-handed training, all encourage associated reactions and therefore contribute to increased spasticity resulting in a worsening of the patient's condition.

(3b) Facilitation of Normal Movement

Inhibition of spasticity
Facilitation of movement
Avoidance of associated reactions

Inhibition of Spasticity. It is therapeutically important to reduce spasticity and to prevent abnormal posture and movement patterns, in order to achieve normal muscle tone. The therapist usually begins to inhibit spasticity proximally in the upper extremity.

The patient is encouraged *to bear weight through his affected side* (Fig 10). This inhibits spasticity of the trunk, arms and legs and makes further treatment easier.

Mobilisation of the shoulder is the basis for the rehabilitation of the arm. For this the scapula is brought forwards and upwards and this is achieved by holding the upper arm in the axilla as well as the medial border of the scapula (Fig 9).

Only the mobilisation of the scapula makes it possible for the arm to cross body midline; if the scapula is fixed, the arm cannot be brought above the horizontal.

The mobilisation of the shoulder girdle is also the prerequisite for achieving rotation against the pelvis. All equilibrium reactions as well as walking need trunk rotation. Hence mobilisation of the shoulder is a 'key point' for all therapeutic facilitations in the rehabilitation of a hemiplegic patient.

'Key points' may also be called 'control points'. Through the change in the position of a 'key point' the control changes over other body parts. The most important 'key points' are proximal — for example, head, neck, shoulder, trunk and pelvis. Through facilitation of these 'control points' spasticity can be influenced distally. With distal 'key points' one can also reduce spasticity proximally — for example, through abduction of the thumb (Figs 18b; 18c; 31; 35b). In order to inhibit abnormal posture and movement patterns in the arm the therapist brings the 'key point' — shoulder — forwards and up.

To inhibit spasticity distally:

The arm is externally rotated, possibly abducted, but more often in forward flexion;
The elbow in extension;
Forearm in supination;
Wrist in dorsiflexion;
Fingers extended and abducted;
Thumb abducted (Fig 10).

To inhibit spasticity the therapist should proceed slowly and avoid abrupt movements. This procedure makes it possible for the therapist to observe and to feel for changes in muscle tone. The patient is also more able to perceive and feel the correct postures and movements.

If the patient is positioned correctly from the beginning and these principles are followed in all treatment, in most cases he will not develop extensive spasticity.

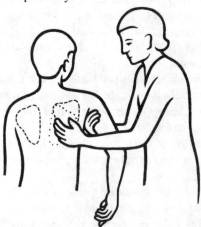

Figure 9. *Position of therapist's hands during inhibition of spasticity in the shoulder.*

Besides inhibition of spasticity there is the possibility of increasing tone in a patient with hypotonus — for example, through tapping, weightbearing and joint approximation. The therapist has to be experienced, having learned these techniques on special courses, in order to avoid increasing spasticity.

Facilitation of Movement. The normalised muscle tone makes facilitation of normal coordinated movement patterns possible. Abnormal movement patterns must be strictly avoided during treatment.

When the hemiplegic patient moves his limbs in an uncontrolled way spasticity develops. To avoid this we choose movement sequences in occupational therapy that work against the abnormal movement patterns.

Example. It would not be therapeutic if the occupational therapist allowed the hemiplegic patient to knit or do any other fine motor task close to the body, with retracted shoulder and with flexion of all the joints in the upper limb. Activities with gross movement sequences, perhaps combined with rotation between pelvis and shoulder girdle, are more suitable.

As long as spasticity is present on the hemiplegic side, only gross motor gripping functions should be practised, because practising fine grips too early — with, for example, knitting and macrame — may increase spasticity.

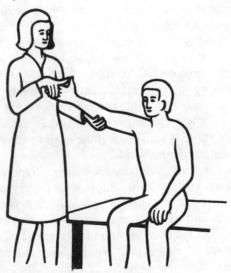

Figure 10. *Reflex inhibiting position of the upper limb. This is also used in preparation for weightbearing.*

The choice of activity should include alternated grip and grip-release, so that an interplay develops and an object is not kept in the hand. During block-printing, for instance, one prints not only with one block but with two alternately (Fig 44).

When treating brain-damaged patients the therapist should look at whole complex movement patterns as well as individual muscle function.

Avoidance of Associated Reactions. The appearance of associated reactions, with increased spasticity, has to be avoided during one-handed training and activities of daily living as well as during general activities. This is an important principle of occupational therapy. If the occupational therapist does not stop associated reactions during activities then she can rightly be accused of worsening the condition of the patient instead of making him better. This kind of occupational therapy, at best, keeps the patient occupied but cannot be called treatment.

Associated reactions can be avoided: through good positioning in reflex inhibiting positions; through weight transfer to the hemiplegic side and weightbearing on the affected arm; and through not allowing uncontrolled activity.

In order to practise function the therapist has to take care that the arm is not just anywhere but that a part of the bodyweight is actually taken through the arm and hand. Weightbearing means actually supporting some part of the bodyweight. This is best achieved if the weightbearing hand is placed near the activity (Figs 11a, b).

By practising the weightbearing function, better awareness of the neglected side is achieved and sensation is facilitated at the same time.

If it is not clear whether or not the patient is taking weight through his arm there are ways of checking this: a piece of foam is put under the patient's palm — only if this is pressed together has the weight been transferred; or if there is active weightbearing through the arm there should be elongation of the trunk.

The aim is not to learn weightbearing over a hyperextended elbow but the flexible control over the elbow joint during weightbearing.

To avoid associated reactions, not only are good positioning, bilateral activities and weightbearing of the affected extremity necessary but uncontrolled activity should also be prevented. Through the controlled activity of the sound hand, abnormal reactions in the affected side may largely be avoided. This means that the occupational therapist should let the patient execute everything slowly and in a controlled way. Step by step, patient and therapist test together how much effort the sound arm is allowed to work with in order to keep the affected arm relaxed and without spasticity.

After the appropriate preparation, the affected arm is placed on the table. This ideal position of the hand is marked with a pen. The patient is reminded that the hand has to stay within the markings and is not allowed to draw back. Activities with the sound hand may then be carried out, first easy ones and then gradually progressing to more difficult ones. During these the patient observes for himself whether or not this ideal position of the paralysed hand is maintained.

In activities of daily living training, one can take the example of dressing. The therapist puts the affected arm into a favourable position so that spasticity will not be increased by the sole use of the sound arm (Fig 10). If the therapist feels an increase in spasticity, the patient's activity is stopped. He should be asked to repeat the same action more slowly and at the same time with less effort. Gradually the patient takes control of the inhibition of associated reactions himself, instead of the therapist. Even if the patient can carry out his activities of daily living by himself, it is only therapeutic if no associated reactions occur.

In the past the occupational therapist was blamed for increasing the pathological patterns of the hemiplegic patient by carrying out one-handed activities using the sound side with no regard for the affected side. With today's knowledge, there should be no cause for such allegations.

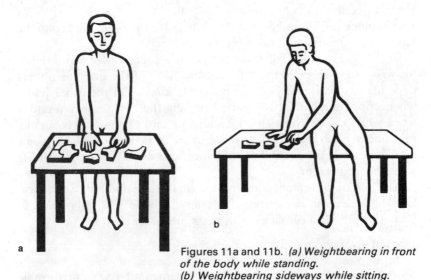

Figures 11a and 11b. *(a) Weightbearing in front of the body while standing.*
(b) Weightbearing sideways while sitting.

(4a) Mass Movements

By the term 'mass movements' one understands a set of complex movements that is so stereotyped that it cannot be altered in any way.

Sometimes a brain-damaged adult may change from a total flexor pattern in all joints in one extremity, to total extension. He cannot, however, bend one joint while a weightbearing one is stretched. The isolated, selected movements that are necessary in daily life are missing.

With such mass movements in the leg, normal walking is not possible. A secure gait calls for the ability to extend the hip with simultaneous knee flexion, as well as dorsiflexion of the foot with flexion or extension of the knee.

Similarly, practical activities cannot be executed with total mass movements of the arm and hand. If the shoulder is forward and the arm extended then the hand can be opened. Even so, gripping in this position is not always possible. If, however, the arm is flexed the grip becomes possible but the hand cannot be opened. Another mass movement of the arm is when in trying to lift his arm the patient uses his whole affected side. Very often he lifts the shoulder girdle with abduction and internal rotation of the arm. The arm, however, cannot be brought into forward flexion. The elbow remains flexed, or will be bent even more, and neither extension nor supination is possible. Wrist or finger movements cannot be carried out (Fig 8).

Selective movements are not necessary only for fine motor activities. Even in opening a window the arm has to be lifted, while the position of the shoulder and elbow has to be maintained at the right height and the hand has to manipulate the window catch.

Real finger mobility will be achieved only if the patient can stabilise his wrist. In both cases the free manipulation of the hand or fingers depends on the stability of the proximal joints. On the other hand, when gripping a hair brush while brushing the hair the distal end is fixed while the proximal joints, shoulder and elbow, carry out the movement. Such individual movements are difficult for the hemiplegic patient because the possibility of fixation and stability in neighbouring joints is not present.

Any lack of movement combinations in the arm and hand is particularly noticeable in occupational therapy because it is impossible to carry out practical activities with mass movements.

(4b) Selective Arm and Hand Function

In order to make distally controlled movements possible favourable positions must be maintained proximally. Good head and trunk control, for example, is the basis for good arm function. Only the secure position and movement of the arm make fine motor movements of the hand possible.

The ability to fix the lifted arm at different heights in order to move elbow and hand independently is the basis for all daily activities like dressing, eating and so on.

During treatment, the occupational therapist has to inhibit and analyse these mass movements to achieve more normal sequences with selective movements. Occupational therapy activities should be chosen so that movements additional to extreme flexion and extension of the arm are practised. While isolated changes of joint positions are demanded, the neighbouring joints should be fixed in their position.

Example. Selective pronation and supination movements in the forearm while turning 'memory' cards (Figs 46; 71).

The treatment in this case is to practise grip function in each position of the arm because this ability is needed in daily life — for example, the therapist offers the pieces of a game from different positions and the patient has to take them. Selective movement within one hand, the individual movements of the fingers and of the thumb for the manipulation of small objects, make great demands on the patient. The therapists have to think about not overworking the patient because an increase in tone may be the result.

At first fine prehension movements are combined, if possible, with gross arm movements. The therapist places the objects that are necessary for the activity in such a way that the patient has to move from one reflex inhibiting position to another. These movement sequences have a positive influence on the fine skilled motor function of the hand.

The aim of treatment should be to overcome and control the abnormal patterns completely so that the distal joints can be moved, controlled and isolated, independently from the position of the proximal joints. Once a patient has mastered these movement combinations, the next treatment goal — automatic movements — can be aimed for.

(5a) Missing Automatic Reactions

Automatic reactions are highly developed motor functions which include equilibrium reactions in all positions, and protective extension.

The term 'equilibrium reactions' means the ability to regain stability at any time quickly and adequately, if the body is not able to compensate with a movement. The static maintenance of a position should not be understood as an equilibrium reaction.

Every movement can change equilibrium and the new equilibrium has to be regained through adjusted activity, i.e. changes within the body (tone, posture, movement, centre of gravity). In order to be able to react correctly a quick adaptation of the muscle tone is necessary. If the weight transfer is only slight, equilibrium is kept only through a change in muscle tone and not with a visible movement. Only large or quick changes in body posture demand movements as compensation to maintain equilibrium.

Protective extension is the ability to support spontaneously with extended hands, by unexpected quick changes of body postures.

Equilibrium reactions as well as protective extension are automatic saving mechanisms that protect from falling or hurting head and face. These reactions are only possible with normal muscle tone and good motor function. They demand the active muscle work of the whole body. It is not possible to execute these consciously because they need to take place very quickly. Patients with only minimal disability — for example, deficits in sensation — or patients who have made good progress often lack only these automatic reactions.

(5b) Facilitation of Automatic Reactions

Equilibrium reactions
Protective extension
Automatic movements

Facilitation of Equilibrium Reactions. If a hemiplegic patient carries out movements only on command during treatment, no automatic functions will be achieved. The patient has to learn to react subconsciously and quickly to the changes in his body. The therapist, particularly the physiotherapist, does this by moving the patient — for example, by pushing him unexpectedly. The patient has to react with movements to regain equilibrium, and to save himself from falling and hurting himself. This has to be practised often and in a variety of ways until it becomes automatic.

In occupational therapy it is even more important to regain equilibrium *automatically* after each change in body posture because any of the activities demand the concentration of the patient — for example, during activities of daily living. Depending on the ability of the patient, equilibrium reactions may be practised either sitting or standing through a gradual increase of the activity radius (Figs 24; 27; 28; 29).

Facilitation of Protective Extension. The preparation and facilitation of spontaneous protective extension can be practised in occupational therapy, as described above. This, however, is more usually concentrated on in physiotherapy.

Facilitation of Automatic Movements. In order to aim not only for conscious movements but also spontaneous automatic ones, the occupational therapist teaches the patient not movements but the 'feeling' for them. She has to make the patient feel the difference between the wrong and the right movements and so give him the sensation for normal ones. The desired direction for a movement is achieved through asking the patient: 'Please, fetch an object from here and another one from over there' — not: 'stretch the arm forward, rotate it and open the hand!'. Two examples follow.

1. The therapist holds the pieces of a game diagonally above and in front of the patient so that he is forced, when trying to get it, to hold his affected arm in forward flexion, external rotation, extended elbow and partial supination (Fig 12).

2. A hemiplegic patient is dropping the pieces of a game into a box on the floor with his elbow bent. Because of the loud noise the patient is startled every time and this results in associated reactions, with an increase in flexor spasticity in the upper limb. Without telling the patient that he should stretch his elbow, he is asked to place the objects as quickly as possible into the box.

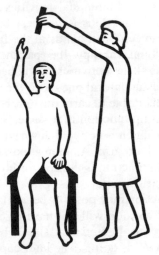

Figure 12. *A rod is held for grasping.*

The desired movement is achieved automatically and, at the same time, undesirable associated reactions are eliminated.

(6a) Lack of Coordination in Both Hands

A hemiplegia disrupts the coordination of the whole body because the fine interplay between both sides of the body is interrupted. As in the early stages, the neglect of the affected side is apparent, as it is later on, even with some good arm and hand function present. If the affected hand is used at all during bimanual activities, it is not moved spontaneously or is slow in relation to the sound hand.

The reasons for difficulties in coordination can be the result of neglect of one half of the body; rotation within the body axis and shoulder retraction; a hemianopia; sensation deficits; or the fact that the affected extremity is only used consciously and for unilateral activities but not for automatic and bilateral activities.

The missing interplay between both hands is a last sign of asymmetry and the lack of coordination of both sides of the body. Also the hand/foot and hand/mouth coordination, as well as the fine coordinated interplay between thumb and finger movements, may be disrupted.

(6b) Useful Coordination of Both Hands

In the early stages the occupational therapist has worked for trunk symmetry through bilateral and bimanual activities and the coordination of both sides of the body. This is the best basis for achieving coordinated interplay between both hands in the late stages.

Early on in occupational therapy the patient has to practise bimanual use of his hands — the activities slowly becoming more and more difficult — as well as unilateral ones with the affected hand. At first the affected hand will be able to carry out only certain holding and supporting actions, until grip function is possible. This means that an object the patient is working on is not held down with a sand sack, but with the affected hand and forearm. As soon as possible, however, the developing weightbearing function is utilised for holding and fixation — for example, when tearing paper.

The regained hand function may possibly be used for holding a fork with a built-up grip, and so food will not have to be eaten with one hand. From the beginning the affected hand should be educated to be a part of what the sound hand is doing. The later coordination of both hands during manual activities demands: good sensation; adequate muscle tone for good fluent movements; the ability to use both hands spontaneously and automatically; and a tuned interplay between both hands.

In the choice of activities, those that make the use of both hands inevitable, are particularly suitable. During these the occupational therapist should ensure that the affected side is not left behind while the sound side moves quickly and spontaneously towards the activity. The treatment aims at simultaneously, bringing forward both hands to the work surface. How this treatment aim can be achieved with sensory deficits is shown in Chapter VII.

The conscious use of the paralysed hand should not be the end goal of occupational therapy. The goal should be the spontaneous automatic use of both hands. Only this ability is useful for the patient in his everyday life.

Even with intensive training, the paralysed hand can rarely be trained to become the dominant one once again. During bimanual activities, tasks are divided in such a way that the sound hand carries out the more complex functions, while the affected hand takes over the easier holding and supporting function.

(7a) Sensory Deficits

Why are sensory deficits as important as the motor deficits of the hemiplegic patient? The reasons are as follows.

Of all the various problems which can be present in the brain-damaged adult, the tactile and proprioceptive disturbances and also disturbances of touch sensation are the ones most closely linked with motor disturbances.

Sensory deficits affect motor function considerably — they can be *the* limiting factor during rehabilitation.

Disturbed motor function can also alter the sensation in the affected limb; although a patient may not have primarily a deficit in sensation, abnormal muscle tone can influence sensation adversely.

This shows how closely sensation and motor functions are linked in the central nervous system, and how they cannot be separated in treatment. This important area of occupational therapy is described in more detail in Chapter VII.

In the initial assessment the hemiplegic patient should not only be tested for motor deficits but also for any deficits in sensation. Sensation may be divided into the following groups: deep sensation; superficial sensation; and stereognosis.

Deficits in deep sensation are those that influence the motor function considerably. Deep sensation gives information about our movements and the positions of our limbs. If this perception is missing, purposeful movements are difficult and the patient has no control over how he moves.

Deficits in superficial sensation make it impossible for the patient to distinguish between different touch sensations: he may hurt or burn himself easily.

Astereognosis is the inability to recognise objects or forms by handling, although tactile, thermal and proprioceptive functions are still intact.

Frequent and noticeable effects of disturbance in sensation result in: non-use of that extremity; neglect of the affected side; danger of accidents; 'bumping' of the arm and hand because the range of movement cannot be judged accurately; and losing objects from the affected hand.

Deficits in sensation may disable a person just as much as deficits in the motor area. If both are combined the result is a doubly severe disability.

(7b) Facilitation of Tactile-Kinaesthetic Perception

Treatment planning should be the result of a detailed sensation test combined with observations of how the patient moves the limb that lacks sensation.

As emphasised, deficits in sensation should never be seen or treated separately from motor deficits because they are very rarely an isolated problem and are more likely to be a sensory-motor problem.

In contrast to patients with sensory deficits resulting from peripheral nerve lesion, the sensory perception of those who have suffered damage to the central nervous system may vary a great deal. The effects depend on body positions and movements, as well as whether or not spasticity is inhibited.

Normalisation of muscle tone is essential as a basis for each treatment, because normal perception is only possible through this. Training of sensation is part of the early stages of treatment and can be integrated into functional activities. Nevertheless, only at a stage of recovery where certain arm and hand functions are possible is it sensible to give priority to this training but it should never be given at the expense of motor training.

In order to experience all the different sensations, the patient requires a variety of stimuli. A range of materials should be chosen — for example, hard, soft, wet, dry, smooth and rough objects.

The patient is encouraged to use his regained functional abilities in combination with his relearned sensation and incorporate them into his activities of daily living.

D. Conclusion

The seven problems which have been described separately above must, of course, be looked at as a whole as they influence each other. If one looks at the range of disabilities of hemiplegic patients, it can be seen that, on one hand, there may be totally normal movement patterns in one patient, while in others some or all of the abnormal patterns are present in varying degrees. Most hemiplegics will, however, fall somewhere between these two extremes.

Each patient has normal as well as abnormal movements, and during the various stages of recovery he could veer towards more normal or more abnormal movements.

The treatment aims at preventing the classical abnormal picture of a hemiplegic patient, and this is possible if the patient is treated early. It is then easier to prevent spasticity and abnormal postural and movement patterns. It is much more difficult to treat a patient with the typical pathology already well-established. Because of their possible influence on each other, where possible all, or at least some of the disturbances should be taken into account simultaneously in assessment and treatment. In addition to motor deficit, for example, sensory deficits, hemianopia, aphasia and change in personality should be considered.

Even so, I have made the motor deficits of the hemiplegic patient and the treatment of them the priority of this chapter, because it is the disabilities arising from these that are the most obvious, and which are also connected with all the other deficits.

Body and spatial perception, and the use and manipulation of objects depend on intact motor function. The ability to perceive information is altered and thereby disabled through a motor deficit. The patient's inability to cope with his surroundings may be explained by these perceptual difficulties.

Other motor problems — for example, shoulder pain, shoulder subluxation, shoulder-hand syndrome, and oedema of the hand — all considerably slow down the rehabilitation of a hemiplegic patient. As these are not the primary problems of the patient, but arise as secondary complications of the condition, they are not described.

IV Assessment of Motor Function

A. Assessment
B. Gross motor function testing
C. Fine motor function testing

The testing in occupational therapy for functions and deficits in the adult hemiplegic patient is not necessarily identical with the testing methods used by the doctor or the physiotherapist. The testing of functional ability in occupational therapy has a practical basis, the application of which is incorporated into later treatment.

A. Assessment

If a patient is referred to occupational therapy with a cerebral vascular accident or a subarachnoid haemorrhage, the therapist cannot plan appropriate treatment on this information alone. Even additional information such as 'hemiplegia' does not say anything about the extent of the disability. It is also important to know whether other deficits exist besides the impairment of motor function.

To establish the degree of disability in a newly referred patient, various areas are tested: motor function; sensation; hemianopia; praxia (for example, the manipulation of objects and tools); orientation in time and space; and independence in activities of daily living.

There are many additional points to consider, but for the initial assessment the testing of the areas described above is sufficient. At the end of the assessment it should be apparent which areas are affected and to what degree.

After the initial assessment, a more detailed assessment of motor function, sensation, perception and independence should follow.

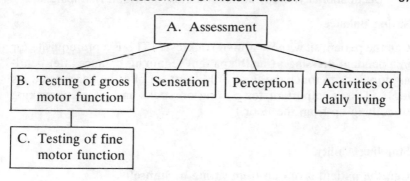

Most occupational therapy departments have a detailed 'activities of daily living' test. Perceptual testing differs between departments and none of these tests are standardised. Even so, with experience and practice, most therapists have learned to assess concentration, memory, spatial relation and praxia.

Sensation and its assessment are described in Chapter VII.

B. Gross Motor Function Testing

The testing of motor function should always correspond with the aims of occupational therapy, i.e. how can a patient apply these functions in all his activities of daily living. In occupational therapy a patient is asked not only whether he can bend and stretch his elbow, but also whether he can lift his hand to his mouth.

It is also important to observe *how* these movements are carried out; it is not strength that counts but the coordination and quality of the movement. An example of this is whether the patient can extend his arm and bring it forwards, or whether he is able to move only within the abnormal pattern with internal rotation and abduction of the shoulder and elbow flexion.

In using our limbs automatically in daily life we depend on the functions of individual muscles, speed of movement or the range of individual joints, but the coordination and interplay between the different muscle groups is a more important factor.

Practical Motor Function Test

Rolling and sitting up in bed are elementary functions of independence and are sometimes prepared for by the physiotherapist.

Sitting Balance

Can the patient sit without arm or backrest? (This is a prerequisite for independent dressing.) Can the patient regain his balance after bending forwards to touch the floor or his foot, or after he has crossed his legs? (This is important for putting on socks and shoes or picking something up from the floor.)

Standing Ability

Can the patient stand up from sitting by himself?
   How is he standing? (a) completely independently? or (b) with help?
   Can equilibrium in standing be maintained while head, trunk and arms are moved? (Important for pulling up of trousers, putting on coat, taking something from a cupboard.)

Mobility

How is mobility possible? (a) with a wheelchair? (b) walking? (c) independently? or (d) with help?
   Can the patient negotiate stairs?
   Is he able to carry light or heavy objects from one place to another?

Function of the Arm

This can vary in lying, sitting and standing, although most testing in occupational therapy is carried out in the sitting position. If the patient has a severe increase in muscle tone, abnormal postural and movement patterns have to be inhibited first before testing can begin because the therapist is interested only in what a patient can do once his muscle tone is normal. This inhibition of spasticity takes time, but is essential and also gives an opportunity for further contact between patient and therapist.
   Even if the motor testing concentrates essentially on the function of the upper extremity, head, trunk and legs are considered at the same time.

Forward Flexion and Abduction of the Extended Arm

How far can the arm be lifted forwards and sideways without compensatory movements of the trunk, or shoulder retraction and internal rotation? (Grip and grip-release of objects in front or next to the body.)

Palm to Different Part of the Body

(1) To right and left knee
(2) To elbow of the opposite arm
(3) To shoulder of the opposite side
(4) To the mouth
(5) On top of the head
(6) To the opposite ear
(7) To the neck
(8) Onto the back (it is sufficient to touch the lumbar region with the back of the hand)

All these movements are essential for independence in personal hygiene and dressing.

Weightbearing

The ability to weightbear backwards, forwards and sideways on the affected arm and hand is important for activities of daily living and may be tested while sitting or standing. While the patient has no active grip function the affected arm, in the weightbearing position, can be used to fix objects which are worked on with the sound hand. The flexion and extension of the elbow, wrist and fingers, pronation and supination of forearm, as well as the opposition of thumb, are not only assessed individually but also in combination. The practical application of these motor functions is also tested.

Grip and Grip-release are Tested

(1) With objects varying in size, weight and texture such as the following examples.

Rubber ball, diameter about 6 cm
Wooden dice, about 5 × 5 × 5 cm
Rod, about 10 cm long, 4 cm in diameter
Piece of wood, about 0.7 cm thick, 7 cm × 7 cm
Large screw
Match
Paperclip

(2) Combining different arm positions such as the following examples.

In front, behind and next to the body

With the arm hanging down
At waist height
On the table
At shoulder height
Above the head
With flexed or extended arm
In pronation and supination

Points to Observe. Is the patient able to grip and grip-release in a controlled way?
Is grip function normal or combined with abnormal movement patterns of trunk and arm?
Are compensatory movements used?
Is the patient only able to grasp the object if it is held out for him?
Are objects picked up accurately from chair or table or do they roll away after the first touch?
Is it possible to pick up a single object out of a bag or box?
Is grip-release slowed down?
Is grip-release possible in certain arm positions but not in others?

Bimanual Activities. During which the coordination of the two hands can be tested are as follows.

(a) Folding and tearing paper. How is the paper held down, with flat hand, fist or elbow?
(b) Fixing a paperclip to these scraps of paper.
(c) Opening and closing a jar (diameter of jar and lid about 7 cm or 8 cm).
(d) Cutting meat with knife and fork.
(e) Peeling an orange.
(f) Winding up a piece of string about 1.50 m long.
(g) Tying a bow.
(h) Assembling a nut and bolt (about 4 cm long and 0.5 mm diameter).

During the assessment of bimanual activities it is important to note which of the hands is dominant, which one takes on more of the holding functions, and whether associated reactions are present.

Assessment of motor function should not be completely separated from treatment. Testing should be part of treatment and observations may be made immediately in treatment sessions. A detailed assessment is the basis for appropriate treatment planning and should from time to time be repeated in order to show progress, regression and whether the treatment plan needs to be altered.

C. Fine Motor Function Testing

Testing for this is done only with patients who have made a good recovery or with people who had only slight impairment of the hand initially. For comparison the activity is carried out with the sound as well as the affected hand.

Finger Dexterity

The dexterity of complex hand functions is assessed on tasks that use the various grip prehensions including opposition of the thumb. Also tested are fine finger combinations such as the following.

Turning, twisting, sorting, picking up, counting out (coins, cards, paper money), holding more than one object in the hand, and releasing one at a time.

Precision grip when picking up small objects (screws, nails, matches).

Control of grip-release in time and space (stacking blocks, throwing balls, quoits, discs).

Movement and Function Speeds

In particular, these concern the testing of diadochokinesis, which is the normal power of performing alternating movements in rapid succession.

The ability to shake a liquid inside a bottle through pronation and supination.

The ability to tap with the whole hand or only with the fingers as, for example, when playing the piano.

The ability to transfer small objects (like marbles) individually, from one container into another while being timed.

The ability to file 100 cards alphabetically (the time taken for this is not only dependent on motor function).

Movements that Need Automatic Reactions

Quick adequate motor movements are necessary when catching a ball; when catching an object which is about to fall on the floor; and during movements that are used in protection or defence — for example, protective extension.

Bimanual Techniques

To test the fine motor coordination of both hands, occupational therapy techniques give plenty of opportunity for observation — for example, macrame, making coil pots and finger weaving. If the sound hand is very active during these techniques the consequent associated reactions that may occur on the affected side make smooth hand function difficult.

During the assessment of fine motor-grip function, speed is not the only important aspect: how the tasks are carried out is also important. Residual abnormal postural and movement patterns may still be present — for example, shoulder retraction. This results in the spastic flexion of elbow and wrist if performing the task is too difficult for the patient. If the leg shows associated reactions during activities with the arm, it should be obvious that that activity is too demanding for the patient at that particular time. Only with normal sensation and normal muscle tone can fine motor assessment be carried out.

In certain occupations such as tailoring, toolmaking, instrument-making and electrical engineering it is important to have detailed assessments and training to help with resettlement back to work.

V Treatment Suggestions During the Different Stages of Recovery

After the therapist has established the different motor problems of the hemiplegic patient (Chapter III), and after the assessment of motor function (Chapter IV), it is possible to plan appropriate treatment.

The time that has passed between the onset of the stroke and referral does not indicate the state of recovery. In order to have some sort of guidance five alternative stages of recovery are described as follows.

A. Stage 1:   No function in arm and hand
B. Stage 2a: Little arm function, no hand function
C. Stage 2b: Grip function in hand, no or little arm function
D. Stage 3:   Arm function and mass flexion in fingers
E. Stage 4:   Lack of fine motor function and diadochokinesis

In each of these stages certain factors have to be taken into consideration.

Degree of spasticity as well as abnormal postural and movement patterns.
Associated reactions.
Lack of equilibrium in sitting, standing and walking.
Disturbance of coordination.
Sensory deficits.
Hemianopia.
Perceptual problems.

A. Stage 1: No Function in Arm and Hand

(a)   Transfers
(b)   The adapted wheelchair

(c)   Positioning of the arm
(d)   Bilateral activities

The patient has a severe paralysis of the arm and hand, either flaccid or spastic. Before concentrating on the rehabilitation of the upper extremity, it is important to focus on the correct sitting position in chair, wheelchair or at the edge of the bed.

(a) Transfers

Without the intervention of the therapist the patient will stand up asymmetrically by using his sound side only. He will push himself up on the armrest or edge of the table or by pulling on an object, which results in the sound side being brought forwards and elongated. Consequently, there is a shortening and backward rotation of the affected side. The weight is mainly on the sound leg. It is essential that the patient be prevented from doing this because it encourages abnormal patterns and increases the tone, which produces associated reactions on the affected side.

Throughout the different transfers — such as bed to wheelchair, wheelchair to chair, wheelchair to toilet and any others that can occur during ADL (activities of daily living) training — it is important that standing up and sitting down be well controlled and become part of the general treatment in all circumstances.

During occupational therapy the patient should always transfer from the wheelchair to a normal chair. This is also psychologically important for the patient because it gives him the feeling of not being confined to a wheelchair for the rest of his life. Sometimes the initial training of transfers is done by the physiotherapist, while in occupational therapy the patient puts it to practical use. Through correct facilitation the patient will gain a 'feeling' for normal movement while standing up and sitting down.

To facilitate standing up the patient needs to 'wriggle' forwards in his seat. This is achieved by weight transfer from one hip to the other and by bringing the legs forward. During this process the therapist has to take care that the affected shoulder as well as the hip are brought forward evenly. The position of the affected leg and foot must be correct before weight can be taken on it. The foot must be flat on the ground and both feet parallel or, if possible, the affected one should be slightly set behind the sound one as this facilitates the weight transfer. Hip and knee should be at right angles and the knee must be over the toes.

In order to keep symmetry, both arms are stretched forwards with hands clasped. In the early stages of treatment the patient's arms may be put round the therapist's waist or neck. Even during later stages of recovery this position is kept to encourage symmetry (Fig 13).

Facilitation has to be such that it enables the patient to bring his weight forward. By increasing hip and knee flexion the whole weight of the body is transferred over the feet. Only when these positions are correct is the patient allowed to stand up. The patient is not allowed to pull on the therapist and the therapist must make sure that she is lifting with her legs and not with her back.

Sitting down is done in reverse order. It should be slow and controlled, stopping at times to make the patient more aware of where his body is.

(b) The Adapted Wheelchair

Most adult hemiplegic patients will be able to walk in one way or another at the end of the rehabilitation. Very often the wheelchair is a means of transport only in the early stages of treatment. Nevertheless, a great deal of time may be spent in a wheelchair and good positioning is therefore of paramount importance. The wheelchair should be correct for the height of the patient. Hip, knee and ankle joints should be at right angles. Detachable arm and leg rests are an advantage. Seats and backrests are very often hammock-like and tend to encourage an asymmetrical sitting posture. To avoid this, firm seats and back-cushions should be used. Suitable ones are those with a plywood base.

Only a few stroke patients can successfully manoeuvre commercially made one-arm drive wheelchairs. The most common form of propulsion is by the unaffected arm and leg. If at all possible, independent

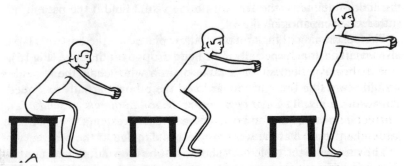

Figure 13. *Symmetrical standing up and sitting down; the patient inhibits his own spasticity through clasped hands.*

mobility in the wheelchair should be encouraged. If, through over-activity of the unaffected side, an increase in tone and associated reactions occur, however, independent use of the chair should be discouraged. Premature use of the wheelchair and walking, as well as unsupervised activities of daily living, will all impede normal posture and movements in arms and legs.

(c) Positioning of the Paralysed Arm During the Day

Outside treatment hours the position of the affected arm is equally important. In the shoulder the dangers are: the weight of the flaccid arm severely pulling on muscles, tendons, joint capsule and the whole shoulder girdle; and spasticity in the shoulder with its resultant abnormal postures usually causing painful shoulders.

Before concentrating on the positioning of the hand, depression and retraction of the shoulder, shoulder subluxation or a painful shoulder have to be dealt with.

If the patient is sitting or standing during the day he should be wearing a pad in the axilla held by a figure of eight bandage. Through the altered position of the humerus in relation to the glenoid fossa, muscles and tendons are not moving normally. By using this support, the swing of the arm is facilitated while walking. The use of a full arm sling should be discouraged because this encourages shoulder retraction, elbow and wrist flexion.

In the early stage the forearm should be placed on a suitable armrest to support the weight. It is not enough just to place the arm on the armrest of the wheelchair — it is too narrow and the arm will fall off constantly; and will not be noticed if sensory deficits exist. If the armrest is widened the arm can be supported, but this type is not long enough to extend the elbow and therefore does not prevent shoulder retraction: neither is the arm within the visual field if the patient has suffered a hemianopia (Fig 14).

The positioning of the arm on a pillow placed on the patient's lap is also unsatisfactory, especially if the hand drops over the edge (Fig 15).

Whether a patient sits at a table or in a wheelchair the shoulder should always be brought forward and the elbow partially extended. *The whole forearm should be on the table and in the visual field of the patient.* If only the hand and part of the forearm rest on the edge of the table, the pressure at the wrist may cause damage to the ulna nerve.

The surface of the table itself should not be too smooth because this makes it difficult to keep the arm in its ideal position. Tables with a lip around them are not advisable, especially for patients with sensory

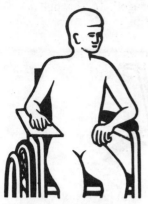 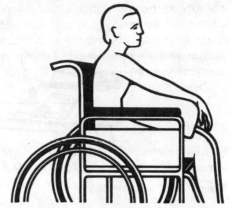

Figure 14. *Positioning of the arm on an enlarged armrest but outside the visual field.*

Figure 15. *Unsuitable positioning of the arm on a pillow.*

deficits, because of the danger of injury. A special wheelchair table for the hemiplegic patient has proved successful (Fig 16).

Materials — 10 mm thick plywood or, better still, perspex as the patient can then keep visual control over the lower half of his body. Both the size of the cutout for the body and of the table will, of course, depend on the individual patient and chair. The table is fixed to the chair by four wooden clips, or by using leather or velcro straps.

If the patient retracts his arm constantly a small dycem mat may be put under it. This prevents retraction. The hand may be raised with a piece of foam to help oedema if present (Fig 17).

Each patient has different needs and the positioning should be adjusted accordingly. A wheelchair table is useful in the early stages but it should be withdrawn as soon as possible in order to encourage

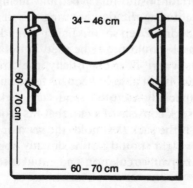

Figure 16. *Wheelchair table, view from underneath.*

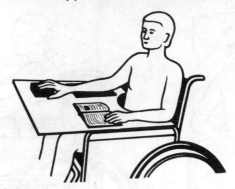

Figure 17. *Wheelchair table in use.*

the patient to sit freely and take responsibility for his arm by placing it by himself on the table.

If the patient's hand becomes spastic, which sooner or later is the case with many hemiplegic patients, it is a mistake to give him a ball to squeeze. Not only does this encourage flexor spasticity in the fingers but it also fails to break the pattern or facilitate grip-release.

Figure 18a shows the foam finger-spreader of the Bobath type. This is preferable to any splint because the resistance of a hard splint only increases spasticity.

The size is about 14 × 14 × 6 cm and the holes are arranged so that the fingers are abducted as well as extended. This has an optimal influence on the flexor spasticity and the position of the wrist (Fig 18b).

Variation of this position can be achieved if the forearm is put into partial supination. The abducted thumb is then on top (Fig 18c).

Not only is the finger-spreader useful when the hand is on the table, but it can also be used for positioning in bed and during the night. If the patient is very active during the day, wearing this device can prevent some associated reactions. Even so, this finger-spreader is not a substitute for treatment and should never be used in isolation.

Only in rare cases where flexor spasticity in elbow and wrist is so severe that the patient is not able to keep his forearm on the table is it possible to use a specially adapted sand-sack to keep the arm in position. This sand-sack consists of a cuff that fits around the patient's wrist; attached to it is the sack that holds the sand or lead pellets. It is important that the weight should not be directly applied to the wrist because this could impair circulation and could also cause pressure sores (Fig 19).

If elbow flexion is combined with a strong tendency to pronation, a

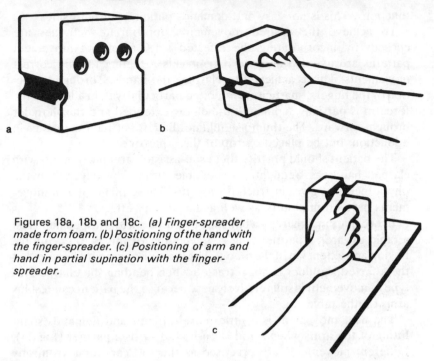

Figures 18a, 18b and 18c. *(a) Finger-spreader made from foam. (b) Positioning of the hand with the finger-spreader. (c) Positioning of arm and hand in partial supination with the finger-spreader.*

cone fixed to the table may be used to keep the forearm in the desired position (Fig 20).

It is always best to position the arm normally on the table without adaptations or aids, but with the patient controlling it himself.

Unilateral activities with the sound hand are often carried out near the edge of the table — for example, when typing. Figure 21 shows the typewriter with an adapted shift control so that capital letters can be operated with the foot. The arm is positioned on a board that is clamped to the table. Through this a symmetrical working posture is achieved.

The different suggestions of how to position the arm while sitting and standing and during leisure time are no substitute for treatment. They complement treatment, however, and should therefore never be neglected.

(d) Bilateral Activities

During Stage 1 the patient has total paralysis of the arm. It is the role of the therapist to mobilise this extremity in order to facilitate returning functions. This is not easy and demands patience on both sides.

To achieve the desired movements appropriate activities are chosen: by incorporating the affected side, abnormal movement patterns are avoided and the patient gets a feeling for the correct movements. This is achieved by clasping the hands. Through adduction of the fingers, spasticity is inhibited particularly if, in addition, the forearm is partially supinated, the elbow extended and the shoulder brought forward. The thumb should not be left between the palms in adduction, but be placed on top of the other one.

The patient should practise these self-assisted arm movements with clasped hands as frequently as possible during the day. Often the physiotherapist gives instructions for this. These bilateral arm movements have an inhibitory as well as facilitatory effect.

In occupational therapy a ball may be pushed with clasped hands on a table towards a partner (Fig 22). The aim of this is to encourage flexion and extension of the elbow. The therapist has to make sure that the affected shoulder is not retracted when bending the elbow. This type of movement is still relatively easy because the patient can rest his arms on the table.

The next movement is a little more difficult and demands slight lifting of the arms when a rod is pushed towards a partner (Fig 23). Different movements are practised as the rod can come from any direction.

Quick and abrupt movements should be avoided because they can increase muscle tone. The affected side needs slow and guided movements in order to be able to recognise them and, later on, repeat them without control.

Sometimes two tables have to be put together to give enough room for larger movements, forwards as well as sideways. It can be stimulating if two patients play together sitting opposite each other at a large enough table, but only if two therapists are present so that any abnormal patterns that occur can be inhibited at once. Group treatment at this early stage is not desirable.

In Figure 24 the rod is moved sideways. If the contact with the rod is not only through the palms but through the forearms as well, quite a difficult movement is demanded of the patient. This also encourages weight transfer, which is important for sitting balance.

All sorts of different remedial games are possible with clasped hands. In Figure 25 a 'number-pushing-game' is shown. Large movements of the arm in all directions are needed to put the numbers in order.

When standing up the patient keeps his hands clasped and uses them

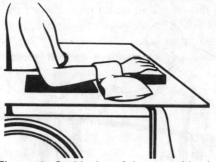

Figure 19. *Positioning of the arm with adapted sand sack.*

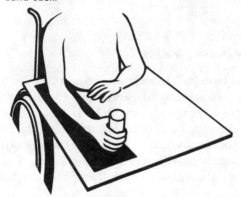

Figure 20. *Positioning of the arm to eliminate pronation.*

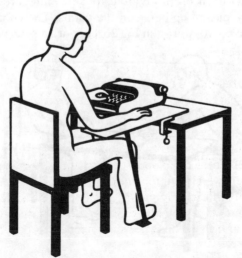

Figure 21. *Positioning of the arm during activities carried out at the edge of the table, e.g. one-handed typing.*

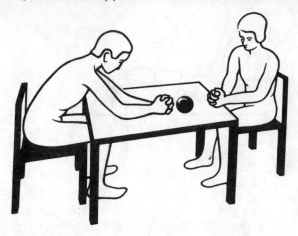

Figure 22. *Bilateral rolling of a ball.*

to push up on the table. Under no circumstances is the hemiplegic patient allowed to use only his sound hand for standing up, as it is difficult to achieve symmetry once lost. If only a monoplegia exists bilateral activities may be carried out standing (Fig 26).

Whether or not activities are generally carried out sitting or standing depends very much on the recovery of the leg. The occupational therapist should liaise with the physiotherapist to establish what is best for the patient.

Bilateral activities with clasped hands are shown in Figs 24–30. Rods or pegs made out of broom handles or dowelling are used as game pieces and are picked up between the palms. The choice of size and position of the board, shown in Fig 26, encourages the patient to make

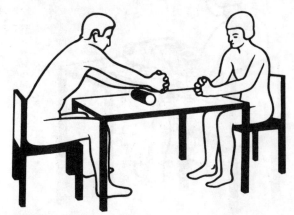

Figure 23. *Bilateral rolling of a rod.*

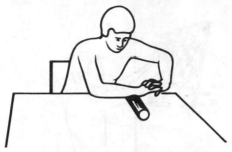

Figure 24. *Bilateral rolling of a rod sideways.*

large arm movements, horizontally as well as vertically. These are important for the mobility of the shoulder. The arm movements desired by the therapist are achieved according to where she places the rods for grasping. The midline should always be crossed because this facilitates shoulder protraction and trunk rotation (Fig 27).

Even so, the therapist should not say to the patient: 'Lift and stretch the arm and rotate the shoulder girdle, please,' but instead say: 'Pick up the rod and put it into the board, please'.

Bilateral activities in the early stages prepare the patient for spontaneous automatic movements (see: Treatment, III (5b)).

If rest periods are required during treatment sessions, it is important that while resting the patient should not be allowed to fall back into abnormal patterns. Both elbows, or at least the affected one, should be on the table and perhaps the head supported by both hands, thus guaranteeing symmetry. These spasticity-inhibiting rest periods are desirable, particularly for overactive patients (Fig 49).

During bilateral activities the therapist should not only work with extended elbows but also incorporate elbow flexion. Part of the treatment aims in occupational therapy is to facilitate arm and hand func-

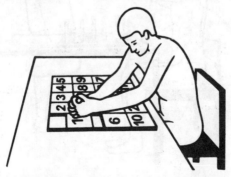

Figure 25. *Bilateral pushing during the 'number pushing-game'.*

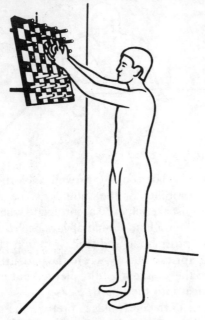

Figure 26. *Bilateral playing of an adapted board game while standing.*

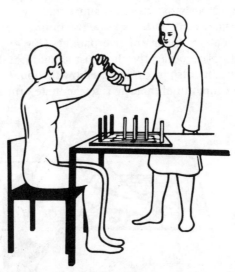

Figure 27. *Bilateral playing of an adapted board game, facilitating shoulder protraction and trunk rotation.*

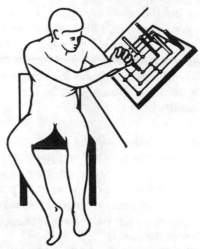

Figure 28. *Bilateral playing of an adapted board game with the hemiplegic leg in an abnormal position.*

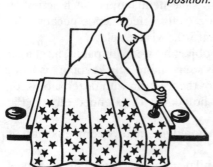

Figure 29. *Block-printing bilaterally.*

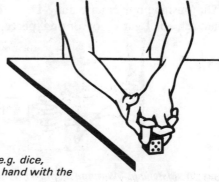

Figure 30. *Picking up an object, e.g. dice, between the fingers of the sound hand with the affected arm in supination.*

tions, but the position of head, trunk and the legs also has to be taken into consideration. This is shown in Fig 28. It is most important that during the activity the affected leg be kept correctly positioned.

As long as the hemiplegic patient is in an abnormal posture, isolated arm and hand movements are useless.

In addition to remedial games creative activities may be used bilaterally.

Examples. Block-printing on paper or fabric; the handles on the blocks are rods so the patient can pick them up between his palms. Ink pads and working surface are positioned in such a way that the backward and forward movements also incorporate the crossing of midline (Fig 29). Batik on paper or fabric; the wax can be applied with a brush or with pastry cutters (with a rod attached) or with cardboard cylinders of different diameters.

With these kinds of bilateral activities one hopes to influence the asymmetrical head position; facilitate equilibrium in sitting; and train compensatory movements for a possible hemianopia. Such activities often make the patient more aware of his affected side because the paralysed arm is always brought into the visual field.

If the patient cannot pick up the object between his palms, he can do so with the tips of the fingers of his sound hand, still keeping his hand clasped. This results in supination of the forearm with flexed elbow, or possibly external rotation of the shoulder with extended elbow (Fig 30).

This type of gripping, however, should not involve compensation of the trunk on the affected side.

Another way of using the hands bilaterally is by having the fingers of the affected hand held in abduction by the sound one. This also has the advantage of inhibiting spasticity (Fig 31).

The pushing movements may be used during matching games or other remedial games or during perceptual testing or training. To

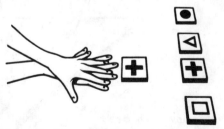

Figure 31. *Matching, with fingers spread, pushing forwards.*

make it easier for the patient, talcum powder is sprinkled on the table. The choice of activities using this hand position is rather more limited than that for the clasped hand position, because the hands are lifted off the table only with difficulty and no grip function is possible. In this position the forearm is in pronation and the palm is in contact with the table. The friction that is created enhances sensation in the hand.

During Stage 1 of recovery the occupational therapist should not wait until the physiotherapist has achieved a particular movement. In order to complement treatment in physiotherapy the occupational therapist uses bilateral activities during which the sound side leads for as long as the affected arm has no function. Through this the patient gains a 'feeling' for movements again.

Even if in severe cases no arm or hand function can be achieved the therapist should aim at the following.

Avoiding contractures and abnormal postures;
Achieving body symmetry or, if possible, a nearly symmetrical posture;
Achieving equal weight transfer with good equilibrium reactions. This is most important for ADL training;
Establishing the patient's awareness of both sides of his body;
Avoiding secondary factors like painful shoulders, back pain or associated reactions.

Bilateral activities contribute greatly towards the awareness of the neglected hemiplegic side and may also help in regaining body scheme. It is desirable for the treatment to be as varied as possible from the beginning. Movements should vary in direction and range, as well as the way in which objects are picked up. This gives the patient a variety of movement experiences.

The patient has to learn to take responsibility for himself so that he can carry over what he has learned during treatment into such activities of daily living as the following.

Polishing a table, sitting or standing (Fig 32);
Dusting;
Cleaning windows;
Using an iron (with guard) (Fig 67);
Using an onion slicer (Fig 70b);
Pushing a chair or table;
Pushing a trolley;
Crossing legs (Fig 69).

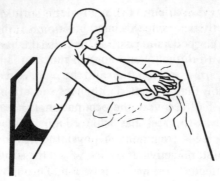

Figure 32. *Polishing a large table, bilaterally.*

B. Stage 2a: Little Arm Function, No Hand Function

(a)   Unilateral activities
(b)   Bimanual activities while using the weightbearing function on the affected side
(c)   Bilateral activities using both arms in the same way

In this second stage of recovery some small movements in shoulder and arm are possible. In some positions the arm can be partially held and moved against gravity.

The development of practical usable movement patterns very often occurs parallel to the development of spasticity and abnormal movement patterns, the latter inhibiting the development of normal movement functions. To prevent the development of hypertonus during treatment, movement sequences that work against these abnormal patterns have to be chosen. Through constant observation and assessment during treatment, the therapist can distinguish between those activities which are developing spasticity and those which are inhibiting spasticity.

As the affected side still has little function — for example, inadequate weightbearing and missing hand function — bilateral activities are still indicated at this stage. Through these the patient experiences a feeling of lightness in his limb. Even so, the sound side is sometimes overused to compensate, thus preventing the affected one from being fully used. In order not to hinder the development of returning functions because of this, more and more unilateral activities are incorporated into the treatment plan.

To achieve coordination of both sides of the body, *bimanual* activities may be used during which the affected side supports and holds while the sound hand carries out the fine intricate movements.

(a) Unilateral Activities

In order to make the first arm movements easier on the affected side the patient receives support from the therapist (Figs 35 and 36).

The slowly improving arm movements are used in Fig 33 for playing skittles. With the fingertips or the back of the hand the ball is pushed forwards with *slow* movements of the arm. It is important to make sure that the movements are not carried out too quickly or abruptly, and that not too much strength is used, because control may be lost and spasticity develop. The skittles are put in a row and the ball has to be pushed in different directions using different movement combinations of the shoulder.

Different pushing activities can also be used, during which the affected hand is held in extension. The remedial games that were carried out bilaterally in the first stage (Figs 22–31) can now be used with the affected arm only.

Matching pairs or completing sequences while working at a table is carried out by using the tips of the fingers while the hand stays flat on the surface (Fig 34). To avoid friction, particularly with people who have perspiring hands, talcum powder may be put on the table or a

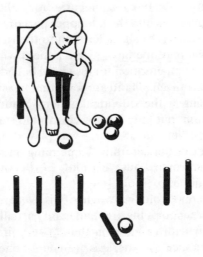

Figure 33. *Playing skittles without grip function.*

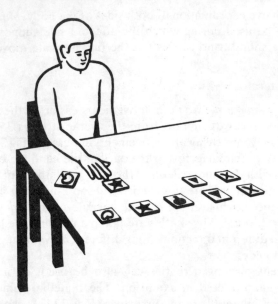

Figure 34. *Matching unilaterally on a table.*

small piece of cloth may be put under the hand. During such activities the weight of the arm is not actively borne because the forearm is still placed on the table.

If the table is large enough the cards or objects are sometimes placed a little bit more to the right or to the left to vary the direction.

Due to spasticity of the flexors, it is easier for right-sided hemiplegic patients to push the cards into the left upper part of the table giving the desirable protraction of the shoulder than to the right. Such activities using the whole width of the table give a patient with hemianopia the chance to practise compensation for his visual field defect. In addition, pushing activities with a flat hand are sometimes easier when sitting or standing, depending on the individual patient. Standing may facilitate functions in the arm, but only if good controlled standing is possible.

The 'number-pushing-game' which was played bilaterally (Fig 25) can now be carried out unilaterally. Depending on regained functions the movements are carried out with a lot, a little, or no help from the therapist (Figs 35a; 35b; 35c).

If the patient cannot hold the weight of his own arm over a period of time the therapist supports the arm and hand partially, and thus makes it easier for the patient to move in the desired directions (Fig 35a). Through this guidance the therapist can feel abnormal movements developing and can inhibit them straight away. At the same time the

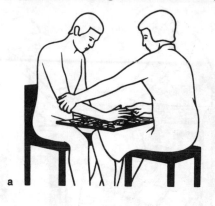

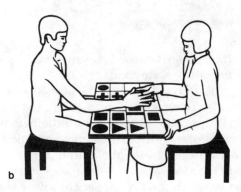

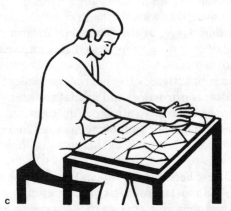

Figures 35a, 35b and 35c. *(a) Playing the 'number-pushing-game' with the therapist's help. (b) Pushing shapes with little help. (c) Using the arm with the hand open, without help.*

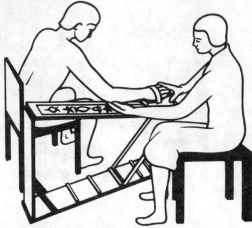

Figure 36. *Downward movement during colouring activity.*

patient is given the feeling of normal movements. As soon as possible any support of the elbow is stopped.

By demanding that the card or object be pushed with the heel of the hand, wrist extension is introduced even before the patient is able to hold the weight of his hand. Often only a little help is necessary to make movements easier — for example, the abduction of the thumb and extension of the fingers by the therapist facilitate good controlled arm movements (Fig 35b.)

The main aim is that eventually the patient will be able to carry out arm movements while extending wrist and fingers independently (Fig 35c). Such arm movements with the hand open also have to be practised during the third stage, at the same time as grip function.

With this type of central nervous lesion it is important to practise *extension* and not flexion.

With these kinds of activities the hemiplegic patient also practises concentration, form construction and spatial concept. These perceptual functions are combined with motor functions.

By using remedial games or suitable techniques, normal movement patterns become more automatic again, and can then be used in all activities of daily living (see Chapter III (5b)).

Activities like these demand a great deal from the patient. He has to carry out controlled movements that are sometimes still difficult for him and at the same time concentrate on the activity. He has to carry out several functions simultaneously, but these demands will face the patient after discharge when he will again have to cope with daily life. This is prepared for step by step in occupational therapy.

Some woodwork activities like sanding and polishing or a form of block colouring (Figs 36; 78) are particularly suitable preparation for function in the arm. The hemiplegic patient should not carry out such activities by himself, but should always be guided by the therapist, particularly in the early stages.

Initially, the angle of the sander is downwards. Through this, extension of the elbow is made easier as the patient works with gravity. During the reverse movement against gravity the therapist should give a helping hand in order to avoid shoulder retraction through elbow flexion (Fig 36).

Fixing the affected hand to any tools with a glove or bandage is wholly unsuitable. This does not achieve active grip function but results in flexor spasticity in the hand. If the affected hand needs to be fixed, for example, onto a sanding or printing block, one has to make sure that wrist and fingers are extended and the thumb is abducted. The various wooden blocks have to be adjusted to the positioning of the wrist. They should have a thin foam lining so that the hand does not glide off. The strap that runs across the back of the hand leaves the thumb free and fixes the hand only lightly (Fig 37).

(b) Bimanual Activities

The wooden block in Fig 38 has a linocut with a piece of velcro attached to it. This has the advantage that blocks with different designs can be interchanged easily. In order to roll the paint onto the design with the sound hand the affected forearm has to be supinated (Fig 38a). The wooden block has rounded edges so that the linocut can be 'rolled' onto the paper using pronation. Through this action, lifting the arm is unnecessary, which is only anyway often possible in the abnormal pattern. If a large piece of paper is used the arm has to be extended in supination in order to reach the corner before printing the design (Fig 38b). The best samples of the prints can be cut out and used to

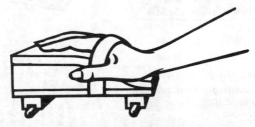

Figure 37. *Positioning the hand on a colouring block.*

make cards (Fig 38c). This type of block-printing facilitates bimanual activity and also the coordination of both hands.

In occupational therapy, movements that are prepared for in physiotherapy are used practically in activities. If the patient has achieved the weightbearing function of his hand in physiotherapy, for example, he can start using this in occupational therapy.

Weightbearing on the paralysed hand can already be incorporated in the early stages of treatment, even if the arm is completely paralysed. The preparation for this is shown in Fig 10 — that is, extension of the arm and opening of the hand. During weightbearing, elbow and shoulder have to be controlled by the therapist. Figure 11b shows lateral weightbearing through the affected side. If the therapist, for example, uses a puzzle where the pieces are placed on the sound side and the frame near the affected side, she practises the following.

> *Weight transfer, facilitation of sitting balance and symmetry* through the forward and backward movements while fetching and placing the pieces.
>
> *Trunk rotation* — rotation of the trunk against the hemiplegic arm because the arm is fixed.
>
> *Associated reactions are eliminated through weightbearing* on the affected side (see also Figs 11a; 11b; 53).
>
> The resulting co-contractions facilitate normal *muscle tone*.

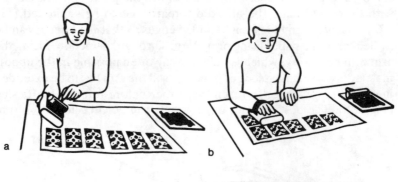

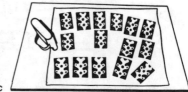

Figures 38a, 38b and 38c.
(a) Lino block-printing with supination.
(b) Printing in pronation.
(c) Finished printed paper.

These weightbearing movements can be beneficial only if the patient sits with a straight back in an upright position. For many patients it is difficult to maintain the weightbearing function with different body positions like side-sitting, four-foot kneeling, sitting and standing, while the rest of the body moves. This has to be practised systematically. With increased motor improvement the patient learns to use this function actively himself.

To achieve coordination of both hands during treatment, an object can now be held with the affected arm through weightbearing (Figs 39; 40). Depending on the condition of the patient, these weightbearing functions may be incorporated into his activity, either sitting, standing, in front or next to the body or, if possible, on an angled high table.

Continued static weightbearing on the arm should be avoided. It is more beneficial to use active weight transfer because each movement and posture change requires the adjustment of muscle tone. One should use techniques where the holding function has to be altered and adjusted quite often.

The treatment aim here is training of coordination and the facilitation of automatic movements.

In later stages of recovery, as well as in this one, the affected hand is used during bimanual activities for the more simple tasks whereas the sound hand is used for more difficult work. If the dominant hand is affected one should not place excessive demands on the patient by forcing him to regain its dominance. If the hand can regain enough function as the non-dominant hand to use it in ADL or at work, then this is satisfactory.

(c) Bilateral Activities

As an addition to the bimanual activities of the first rehabilitation

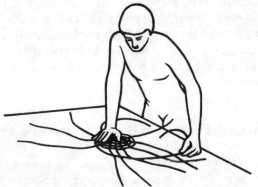

Figure 39. *Sisal or cane weaving; weightbearing on the affected arm.*

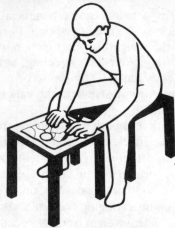

Figure 40. *Drawing around templates, weightbearing in sitting.*

stage, the therapist can now choose bilateral activities during which the returning arm function is used — for example, the arm has to be brought into supination while carrying a big bowl or box with both hands. These movements are also needed for the enlarged span game. The inside rods need not be straight all the time because, by using angles, external rotation and supination of the affected arm are practised (Fig 41).

To avoid associated reactions during bimanual or bilateral activities, planning movement sequences through suitable activities is necessary. The danger is that during an activity where both hands are needed the sound hand is used spontaneously and quickly while the affected one is left behind. This results in the backward rotation of the hemiplegic side and retraction of the scapula.

Additional associated reactions contribute to the typical abnormal pattern of the arm. The increase in tone makes it difficult for the affected hand to get near to the object. This is made easier if the affected hand is used first or if both hands are brought towards the object simultaneously. The therapist can observe that such symmetrical movement sequences with both arms facilitate the active movements of the affected one.

C. Stage 2b: Grip Function in Hand, No or Little Arm Function

If the patient cannot lift his arm adequately, however, certain grip functions are possible. With some hemiplegic patients, Stage 2b follows Stage 1 of recovery, which means that recovery occurs distally to

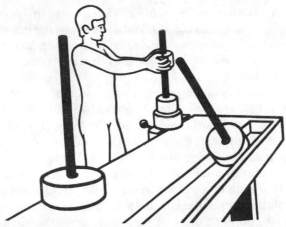

Figure 41. *Enlarged span game, changing of large discs bilaterally.*

proximally, grip function develops before arm function.

A functional hand which the patient cannot bring to a point where it can be used is of little value to him. The ability to stabilise proximal joints is necessary to make distal movements possible and useful.

For useful Hand Function one needs Stability in Shoulder and Elbow. Shoulder–arm–hand form a functional unit which cannot be separated. This means that at this stage the therapist has to concentrate on developing the whole arm function. Part of the treatment plan should also be: bilateral activities as in Stages 1 and 2; weightbearing through the affected arm; using the affected arm for pushing with the weight of it partially supported; and bimanual activities.

If the patient regains the ability to hold an object in his hand, the occupational therapist has to judge whether or not this is done with pure flexor spasticity. The abnormal movement pattern with internal rotation, flexion and pronation are easier for the patient than external rotation, extension and supination. This means that holding an object is easier than letting go of it.

For Good Grip Function one needs the Ability to Control the Opening and Closing of the Hand. A patient has to have the ability to let go of an object in the desired place and at any time. In order to make this possible, the occupational therapist has to plan different goals in the different stages of recovery that facilitate grip and grip-release.

If lifting the arm is still impossible, proximal movements may be used. The hand can be brought to the front of the body while the arm is hanging down, using circular movement in the shoulder.

When playing skittles, as shown in Fig 33, without grip function, the ball can be held in the hand (Fig 42). The diameter of the ball is about 6 cm which seems to be the most suitable size for first grip functions. The balls can be given to the patient from all directions (front, right, left and next to the body).

The same size ball can be adapted as a piece of a game. As the patient is not yet able to bring the arm above the horizontal, the game is not played on a standard table but on a low one (Fig 43).

Two blocks used alternately during fabric printing enable the patient to practise grip and release in succession. Additionally, two different kinds of blocks may be used— for example, one with a vertical handle, the other with a round or horizontal one. The printing has the same effect as weightbearing on the affected arm; it achieves the co-contraction of agonist and antagonist of the whole arm, the simultaneous contractions of flexors and extensors (Fig 44).

D. Stage 3: Arm Function and Mass Flexion in Fingers

In this stage of recovery the arm can be lifted above the horizontal and gross motor functions are possible. Use in normal activities is still difficult for the hemiplegic side.

The occupational therapist should remember that as the sound side is much more capable of doing things, a tendency remains to neglect the hemiplegic side. To facilitate the abilities of the affected side, overactivity with the sound side should be avoided.

During the course of rehabilitation the patient develops not only useful functions but also some abnormal movement patterns. The latter must be inhibited so that the former can be facilitated.

Improvement of hand function is best achieved with the simultaneous improvement of arm function. The opportunities for varied grip movements in all positions of the arm are shown in the use of a game (Figs 45a; 45b). The solitaire board is fixed on a hydraulic table at such a height that the patient can just reach it in elevation. Such tables, which are adjustable in height and plane, are absolutely essential in occupational therapy.

The following movement sequences are shown in Fig 45a. A patient with a right hemiplegia picks the pieces out of a box placed on the floor in front of him, or to his right side. By placing the chair at a certain angle to the table the hemiplegic arm has to cross not only into contralateral body space but trunk rotation is also achieved when placing the piece onto the board.

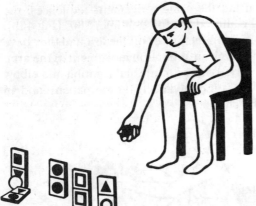

Figure 42. *Playing skittles with early grip function.*

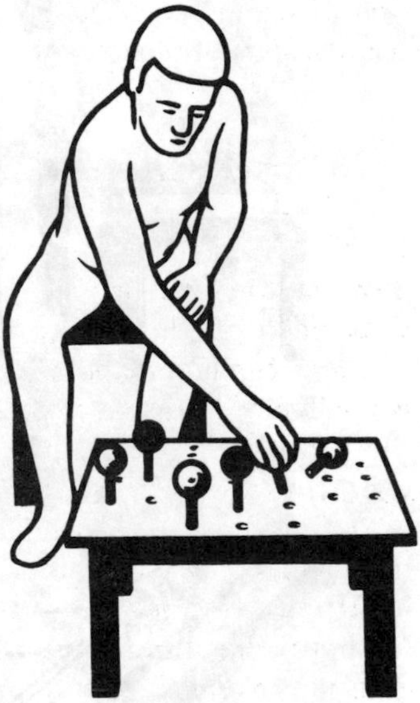

Figure 43. *Practising early grip functions on a low table.*

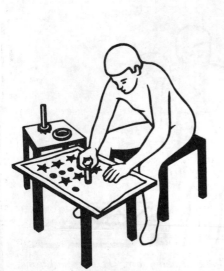

Figure 44. *Block-printing with different handles.*

To avoid fatigue from using the same movement sequences, the position of the chair may be altered by, for example, 180° (Fig 45b). Now the right hand has to pick up the pieces on the left and they have to be placed on the board through an abduction movement of the arm. If the latter movement is carried out with internal rotation and elbow flexion, however, the activity is too advanced for the patient, and an easier movement should be chosen.

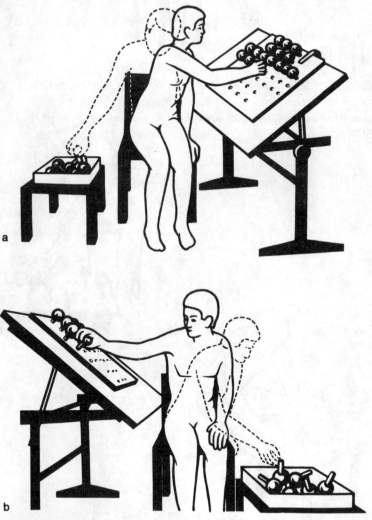

Figures 45a and 45b *(a) Combined training of hand, arm, shoulder and trunk, using a remedial game. (b) Variation of the use of a remedial game through different positioning.*

Excessive Demands Easily Lead to Abnormal Movements. With the Help and Guidance of the Therapist These Can Be Avoided. To achieve the desired treatment goal the therapist either asks the patient to pick up low and place high (Figs 26; 28), or pick up high and place on a low positioned board (Fig 43). With these enlarged remedial games one can practise the gross motor grip functions with different adapted pieces. (See also Chapter IX, treatment media, section D.)

Upgrading may be achieved not only by changing the shape of the pieces of the game, but also by how the patient is asked to grip them.

At the beginning the objects are held in a position so that the patient can grasp them easily.

The next step is that an object positioned anywhere on table, chair, or floor is grasped by the patient. This demands good automatic grip function because the object may roll away if the first attempt is not successful. In addition, the hand has to be brought through pronation and supination, as well as wrist movements, into the appropriate functional positions.

Taking the rods from their holes in the board (vertical) is an added difficulty.

Choosing one object from several in a box is much more difficult for a hemiplegic patient than choosing objects that lie individually, because the grip has to be well judged, coordinated, precise and accurate.

If the patient is asked to pick something out of a bag it is more difficult because vision is excluded (Fig 64).

There are other adapted games besides board games. Wooden blocks (8 × 8 × 4 cm or 6 × 6 × 2 cm) are covered with velcro. The pieces of some matching games or puzzles have the other half of the velcro attached and are interchangeable — for example, one can play 'Memory' in this way practising pronation and supination (Figs 46; 71).

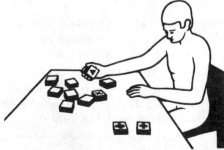

Figure 46. *Grip and grip-release in pronation and supination.*

All these remedial games used in treatment have the advantage that movement sequences can be varied. Apart from the pure motor function, compensation for a hemianopia, spatial thinking and other perceptual functions are also practised. Movement sequences may also be practised using some functional activities as in Stage 4. Some examples are given below.

Woodwork. This demands a practical application of all returning arm and hand functions when sawing, planing, sanding, drilling and assembling the parts.

Fabric Printing. This was carried out in the third stage on a low stool (Fig 44) and might now be done on a more or less vertical table. The inkpad is positioned lower in order to achieve forward and backward movement of the arm. According to the recovery of grip function different block adaptations may be used.

Weaving. Weaving places different demands on the hemiplegic patient. These are: spatial thinking; compensation of a hemianopia; observation of the right sequence of the work process; frequent grip and grip-release in different positions; varied gross motor sequences for the arm; and coordination of arms.

Even so, weaving has one unsuitable movement for the hemiplegic patient — that is, the beating down of the weft with the heddle. This movement leads to abnormal patterns in the arm because it is carried out with elbow flexion, and often with shoulder retraction. For this reason it is advisable to turn the table loom by 180°. Now the beating down demands extension movements of the arm (Fig 47).

E. Stage 4: Lack of Fine Motor Function and Diadochokinesis

At this stage, the patients treated are either those who had only a mild disability to start with, or those who have made a great deal of improvement. These patients have good arm function and are able to grip and grip-release. They are not yet completely ready for all activities of daily living or for a return to work. The final fine motor, as well as quick reaction movements and dexterity are missing, but it is often not easy to treat such a patient effectively because the main reason for this functional deficit in fine skilled prehension movements may lie elsewhere.

To succeed with treatment at this stage it is necessary to observe in

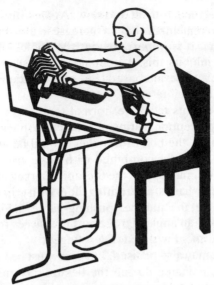

Figure 47. *Weaving on a table loom turned 180°.*

detail, and analyse exactly, what the patient's actual problem is. This can be achieved by letting the patient use skilled finger movements with different body positions and movement combinations — for example, sitting, standing, with arm extension or flexion, with external or internal rotation, with supination and pronation, in contralateral or ipsolateral body space, with different head, shoulder or trunk positions. Through this the therapist can see where fine manipulation is more successful, and in which combinations it is difficult. The results of this analysis form the basis for the treatment plan. These are the possibilities:

(a) instead of building up strength, coordination training with normal muscle tone;
(b) distal improvement through treatment of the proximal joints;
(c) opposition of thumb;
(d) diadochokinesis and automatic reactions; and
(e) other disabilities that can influence fine skilled movements.

(a) Instead of Building-Up Strength, Coordination Training with Normal Muscle Tone

Even at this advanced stage when no spasticity is evident, a small increase in tone can hinder normal reciprocal innervation. Through this, movements become difficult and slow. Again, even at this stage of recovery one has to remember that an increase in tone in the arm takes place in the flexors. It is important that the choice of occupational therapy activities inhibits this. Under no circumstances should the strength of the flexors be increased, but coordination of movement sequences should be facilitated.

Large arm movements facilitate normal tone and also fine motor functions. During perception testing or problem-solving sessions using matches, for example, the box of matches should be at a distance so that grip and grip-release is combined with large arm movements.

To achieve normal muscle tone the therapist can select different arm movements with open hands, alternating them with grip function of the fingers — for example, the 'number-pushing-game' in Figs 25 and 35a, 35b, 35c, is played at an angle. To prevent the pieces from falling the patient has to hold them with extended fingers.

Vertical sanding may also be used, but care must be taken to ensure that resistance is eliminated during the flexion movement.

Macrame is an unsuitable activity because the threads are always pulled tight with the arms in flexion.

At this stage, some patients complain of not having enough strength in arm and hand. This is not so, however: it is more a deficit of coordination between agonist and antagonist and is the result of the lack of reciprocal innervation.

Example. A patient with right-sided hemiparesis, a bricklayer by trade, made such good recovery after a few months of treatment that a work trial was carried out. At the end of the first week, however, the patient complained about not having enough strength to do his work. He was right-handed and wanted to use his trowel with that hand. I visited him at his place of work in order to see what was happening.

I found that his movements were considerably slower, more difficult and awkward than those of his colleagues. He lacked the quick, skilled switch from pronation to supination which is used to get the mortar onto the trowel and then onto the bricks. By the time my patient had his mortar on the bricks it was already too hard to level out. The strength to hold his trowel was not missing; on the contrary, he was holding it so tightly that it was difficult for him to let it go.

The light controlled grip when making a fist is the one necessary for manipulating a handle in the hand. For the different movements of his work, he needed to be able to hold the trowel in different ways and he was unable to carry out this particular change of grip. Through one muscle group becoming too dominant the antagonists could not fulfill their function. This was not due to loss of strength but to a deficit in coordination.

To rehabilitate this patient effectively one had to practise harmonious, quick, skilled movement sequences which are possible only with normal muscle tone. This is further proof that a patient with a central nervous lesion does not lack strength but the quality of movement, and also that the therapist should practise normal coordinate movements and not try to build up strength.

(b) Distal Improvement through Treatment of Proximal Joints

If fine motor movements are deficient and slow the therapist may take into account only the distal areas like wrist and fingers, thereby overlooking the fact that the problem could lie proximally.

Examples. Asymmetrical position of head and trunk with one-sided weightbearing during standing and sitting, shortening of the affected trunk, rotation within the body axis and lateral flexion of the neck.

Reasons for the deficit in skilled movement may lie in the shoulder area — for example, if the shoulder is retracted and internally rotated. Sometimes the shoulder is held too far up or too far down. Movement limitations within the shoulder always impair fluency of movement sequences of the functional unit of arm and hand. A painful shoulder is very often responsible for that.

Most activities need continuous movements. If the arm is raised simultaneous movements of the shoulder girdle are necessary, and if the fingers are used to pick up an object the wrist has to adjust at the same time. Without this fluency of movement in the arm it is not possible to write because, despite good hand function, the shoulder and arm are not moving.

Other activities demand the holding and placing action of the proximal joints so that distally skilled movements can take place. The holding and placing ability may be insufficient and may influence the fine motor skills negatively.

Poor hand function may be the result of insufficient supination.

It is impossible to use the fingers in a skilled way if the wrist has inadequate holding or movement functions.

To achieve functional improvement distally, the therapist has to treat the arm as a functional unit. While facilitating correct movements proximally in head, shoulder and trunk she automatically encourages distal functions.

The occupational therapist chooses movement sequences that work against the abnormal patterns which at the same time enable the patient to move without pain— for example, if the patient complains of shoulder pain because he is retracting his scapula, the therapist uses activities whereby he frequently has to cross the body midline. Through trunk rotation and the protraction of the scapula, normal muscle tone proximally to distally is facilitated, thus promoting skilled motor functions. An object is picked up in contralateral space from a table, and if the therapist holds something further out on the other side external rotation and supination are achieved.

To achieve fluency in writing, shoulder and arm functions have to be encouraged. The therapist can also ask the patient to draw a horizontal line with or without a ruler. Unbroken wavy lines are also good practice, as is the polishing of a table or a blackboard. Use of the pen with continuous arm movement is also encouraged while playing dominoes. This involves pushing the pieces with the pen from the bottom left-hand corner, using rotation and protraction, to the upper right-hand corner, using elevation and extension.

If weightbearing against a wall or a vertical table is difficult, the patient will be unable to hold a picture to the wall until it is secure. Inadequate proximal holding and placing functions are responsible for this. Again, the activity shown in Fig 47 may be used vertically. The affected hand has to hold the wooden blocks so that they do not fall down. A more difficult activity would be making a collage on a cork wall, because the patient has to hold the picture first and then fix the pieces with drawing pins.

Block-printing against an angled surface also facilitates these holding and placing functions. If the print gets smudged downwards this means that the holding function in elevation is insufficient. If the print is smudged sideways this is a sign of abnormal internal rotation of the shoulder, or abnormal pronation of the forearm.

Supination can be promoted with games like 'Memory' or 'Reversi'.

Wrist extension must be practised in order to achieve good fine finger manipulation.

(c) Opposition of Thumb

It is often possible for the thumb to oppose to the first and second finger but not to the fourth and fifth finger. Because of this, fine finger manipulation is impaired. With insufficient opposition it is difficult to pick up thin objects like cards, discs or pins. Opposition to each finger is practised, firstly with thick and large objects and then with thinner ones. Different techniques may be used.

(d) Diadochokinesis and Automatic Reactions

Small increases in tone and traces of abnormal posture and movement patterns are often reasons for the lack of diadochokinesis and delayed or missing automatic movements.

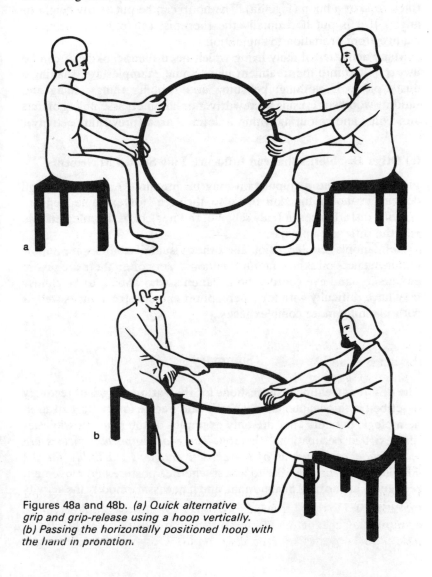

Figures 48a and 48b. *(a) Quick alternative grip and grip-release using a hoop vertically. (b) Passing the horizontally positioned hoop with the hand in pronation.*

The basis for these quick movements is a normal and adjustable muscle tone and this is needed for playing any ball, quoit or balloon game. The therapist can practise these by rolling tennis or squash balls on a long table towards the patient which he then has to catch unilaterally, bilaterally or alternatively with his left or right hand, sometimes in pronation and sometimes in supination. He has to return them in the same manner.

Rapid change of movements may be practised with either a rod, a thick rope or a hoop (Fig 48a). The hoop can be put at any height or angle. If it is put horizontally the therapist can practise the quick change from pronation to supination.

Many activities of daily living which need diadochokinesis can be incorporated into the treatment plan. Some examples are: shaking a dusty piece of clothing; polishing and rubbing things; filing and sanding woodwork; using a screwdriver or hammer; assembling of nuts and bolts; and colouring within a defined area (prewriting activity).

(e) Other Disabilities that can Influence Fine Skilled Movements

Fine skilled hand manipulation may be impaired not only through deficits in motor function but also through, for example, sensory deficits, disturbances in body scheme, the neglect of the affected side and the different apraxias.

Hemianopia, double vision and other visual disabilities are important influences on skilled motor functions. Very often there are severe deficits in hand-eye coordination. Patients who appear to be clumsy may have difficulty with form perception and construction, as well as with planning more complex tasks.

Summary

The different treatment suggestions for the various stages of recovery described in this chapter are not a 'fail-safe' recipe for treating an adult hemiplegic patient. They are only examples of the many possibilities that exist in occupational therapy. *The most important factors are observation and analysis of the chosen activity's suitability for the individual patient.* One has to assess whether posture and movement sequences are normal or abnormal, and if necessary modify the activity accordingly.

VI Bilateral Group Activities

The kind of occupational therapy with the hemiplegic patient described in the previous chapter is possible only on an individual basis, because the therapist has to adjust treatment to the individual patient's needs. With some longstanding patients, however, one should consider whether treatment in a group using bilateral activities would be an appropriate complement to the individual programme.

Non-bilateral activities are suitable only if there are enough therapists present to control them.

Indications for Group Treatment

To intensify and complement individual treatment.

To stimulate patients who lack motivation. Hemiplegic patients are sometimes more inclined to participate in their treatment if they see others with the same disability doing so.

To avoid setbacks and worsening of the condition during acute staff shortage, such as holiday times when individual treatment time may be minimal.

As a transition from individual treatment to 'self-treatment' after the patient has been discharged. Suggestions for a home programme may be given.

For maintaining progress made with older patients in long-term care — for example, nursing homes, geriatric wards or day centres.

If the hemiplegia is longstanding and improvement is minimal, there is the danger in the chronic stage that abnormal postural and movement patterns increase, resulting in contractures, especially by inactive patients.

This kind of maintenance therapy, which has to continue for years, is, I think, possible only in a group.

Contraindications for Group Treatment

Severely disabled patients who lack sitting balance and have marked abnormal movement patterns and spasticity that needs the constant control and help of the therapist.

Patients of whom very little can be demanded — for example, those who lack concentration, are labile or drowsy.

Patients with severe receptive aphasia where a group is too frustrating. Even so, talking in a group can be stimulating for aphasic patients.

Patients who are unsuitable in the group for any other reasons.

The indispensable individual treatment sessions, particularly at the beginning but also throughout the various stages of recovery, cannot be replaced by group treatment.

Principles of Group Treatment

A group that is conducted by one or two therapists should have four to six patients at most.

All participants should transfer from their wheelchairs to a normal chair if possible. Only if a patient has a severe lack of sitting balance should he stay in his chair (for safety reasons).

The patients are positioned in a circle or around a table. The therapist usually has no fixed place as he/she has to go round to help and correct positions.

The choice of activity has to be adjusted to those present. If competition is used, all participants should have a fair chance. The type of games where success is assured should therefore involve luck rather than depend on ability in movement or speech.

Activities are preferably bilateral, whereby the patients inhibit their own spasticity by clasping hands.

All participants should be able to adopt a symmetrical posture which includes control over the position of the legs.

To avoid shoulder retraction the therapist should make a rule that during rest periods both elbows whether flexed or extended should be on the table (Fig 49).

Activities should be chosen in such a way that the movement sequences include forwards and upwards, as well as right and left movements.

Social contact between the participants should be encouraged. The

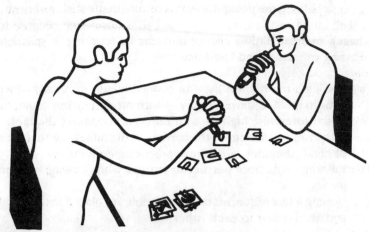

Figure 49. *Symmetrical position of trunk and shoulders when working as well as during rest periods, e.g. when playing 'Memory'.*

therapist sometimes has to initiate conversation. During this time the clasped hands may be put and kept either on or behind the head. As a change music may be used for group activities.

Examples of Bilateral Activities within the Group

(1) Rods or balls may be pushed towards each other on a suitably large table.

(a) Pushing a ball with clasped hands, forwards and sideways while the forearms are on the table (Fig 22).
(b) Catching the ball between the forearms (Fig 23).
(c) With the forearms pronated, elbows flexed and slight abduction and internal rotation of both arms, the palms are put onto the ball. By rolling the ball via the palm and forearm it is passed to the next person (Fig 24).
(d) Rolling the ball through or around obstacles, or hitting the skittles that are placed in the middle of the table.

There are many other variations, and one can play with one or more balls. As well as motor function, attention and reaction ability, and compensation for a visual field defect are practised. If the speed is increased, the therapist has to be careful that movements do not become abrupt and hasty, which always leads to increased spasticity.

(2) Using a balloon the group has to make sure that it stays airborne. A beachball might be used, but a normal ball is unsuitable because it is too heavy and can lead to abrupt movements resulting in spasticity.
(3) Passing objects round the table.

    (a) Passing a rod bilaterally with clasped hands; vertically — with arms in midline; horizontally — with pronation and supination of the forearms; high — with raised arms; under the table — with vision excluded; at the corners of the table — with rotation of head, shoulder and trunk, practising equilibrium.
    (b) Pushing cards from partner to partner while playing matching games.
    (c) If using a technique, material and tools are placed in the middle and are pushed to each other.

(4) Other games — for example, 'Dominoes' or 'Colour Tactics'.
(5) Board and dice games. The board games are adapted by using pegs so that they can be grasped bilaterally and be put into holes. The dice are thrown as in Fig 30 — for example, 'Snakes and Ladders', 'Ludo'.
(6) 'Memory'. Any pair (pictures, numbers or any other) may be used. Each card has a paperclip attached. The cards are turned by using a piece of dowelling that has a magnet attached at the bottom (Fig 49).
(7) Painting, block-printing as a group activity; brushes, pens or blocks with handles attached are again held with clasped hands. A large piece of paper may be used, but fabric is also suitable (see also Fig 29).

Further examples and variations of bilateral group activities are left to the imagination of the therapist.

To end this chapter, I would like to emphasise again that the treatment of a hemiplegic patient is only exceptionally carried out in a group. The different disabilities of a brain-injured adult demand individually adjusted treatment to suit the individual's needs.

VII Sensory Deficits

A. Function and Quality of Sensation

(1) Subdivision of sensory functions
(2) Sensation and body scheme
(3) Sensory deficits of the foot
(4) Facial paralysis
(5) Hypersensitivity to tactile stimuli

Besides hearing, tasting, smelling and seeing, sensation is another sense that is made up of different modalities. The hand, as well as lips and tongue, is rich in sensory nerve endings. It is capable of gripping, lifting, gross as well as fine movements, being used in gesture; in short, it is applied to the most diverse manipulations. As long as these various complex activities function normally, one hardly ever thinks that such activities are made possible only through these additional sense modalities.

Depending on the area and the extent of the cerebral vascular accident, sensory deficits may appear alongside motor deficits, resulting in a more complex disability for the hemiplegic patient. Even if they occur in isolation they influence motor functions considerably.

A deficit in sensation is a severe disability and may implicate the whole side of the body. The effect on the upper limb is particularly disabling.

(1) Subdivision of Sensory Functions

(a) Deep (proprioceptive) sensation
(b) Superficial (exteroceptive) sensation
(c) Stereognosis

Tactile-kinaesthetic perception is a network of different sensory influences and activities. One sense modality complements and supports the other. Through this, the central nervous system receives accurate information from the peripheral areas.

Understanding of the different types of sensation is useful for the therapist, because this helps in the assessment and the establishment of a treatment plan.

(a) Deep (proprioceptive) Sensation This modality refers to the position and movements of the body, and is sensed by receptors located deep in the body tissues, (muscles, tendons, periosteum and joints). They give the appreciation of movements and positions of the body and limbs in space, as well as judgement of weight. Information regarding the correct tension within each muscle is necessary for movement control.

Through these receptors the central nervous system receives continuous proprioceptive stimuli which are followed by an appropriate motor response, which may be either stimulating or inhibiting. A deficit in the area of deep sensation is therefore always a sensory-motor disability.

(b) Superficial (exteroceptive) Sensation The exteroceptive modalities are sensed by receptors located in the skin and include touch, pressure, warmth, cold and pain. This information is relayed to the appropriate areas in the central nervous system.

(c) Stereognosis Stereognosis is the ability to recognise three-dimensional objects by touch. This seems to be a combination of deep and superficial sensation. Intact stereognosis makes it possible to identify the surface of an object, through touch, as well as its shape, size and consistency. Deficits in the area of superficial as well as deep sensation may lead to astereognosis, which can also be called a tactile-kinaesthetic sensory loss, as touch as well as kinaesthetic perception is disturbed.

(2) Sensation and Body Scheme

Not only are sensation and motor functions closely linked, but other perceptive functions of the brain are also interconnected and overlap with them.

A deficit in deep sensation cannot be separated from a disturbance in body scheme. This is a term used to denote the way in which a person perceives the position of, and the relationship between, the different parts of his body. This is important for normal movement.

Examples. Finger location through light touch or pressure. If the patient shows no reaction to either, it is assumed that a deficit in sensation is present. If, however, the patient names his fingers incorrectly, a disturbance in body scheme has to be considered.

In order to initiate motor postures one needs not only good motor functions and proprioception but also intact body scheme.

During ADL training the arm of the patient may get stuck in his clothes. If he has pure sensation problems he will be able, with visual control, to resolve the problem. A patient with body scheme disorder, however, is unable to help himself in this situation, because he has no reference to his body and his clothes.

To complete the picture three other areas of sensory deficits will be mentioned but not considered in detail, because they do not fall solely into the area of occupational therapy.

(3) Sensory Deficits of the Foot

The ability to feel is present throughout the body but varies in intensity according to the area. Tactile-kinaesthetic ability is less developed in legs and feet than in the hands. Occupational therapists are more often concerned with arms and hands but should not forget that the patient may also have deficits in his feet, which for example can make it difficult for him to keep his heel on the ground during activities.

Disturbances in proprioception in the foot make walking insecure, particularly on uneven ground, make negotiating stairs difficult and impair the ability to drive, because the patient finds it difficult to press the pedals accurately.

Physiotherapists incorporate these deficits into their treatment programme and the occupational therapist can help by letting the patient stand correctly weightbearing during activities. One has to take precautions to avoid burns and injury to the foot, particularly during kitchen activities.

(4) Facial Paralysis

Sensory deficits of the face are often combined with motor lesions. While eating, injuries to the face, and particularly the mouth, have to be avoided. If sensation is not present in the lips the patient should never be given a 'Nelson knife' for both cutting and eating but he should be encouraged to cut with the knife and then eat with a spoon. Missing sensation in the lips can also lead to inadequate lip closure which, in turn, results in loss of saliva, messy eating and slurred speech.

Treatment of the face is also sometimes undertaken by physiotherapists or speech therapists. Occupational therapists incorporate the facial treatment into their eating training.

The facilitation of lip closure, tongue, chewing and swallowing movements are helped by sensory stimuli like icing and brushing.

(5) Hypersensitivity to Tactile Stimuli

This is relatively rare in an adult hemiplegic patient, compared with children suffering from cerebral palsy. The patient shows an increased motor reaction to a tactile stimulus—for example, he displays a kind of grasp reflex if an object touches the appropriate area in the palm. With such tactile hypersensitivity present, the therapist plans a desensitisation programme and starts with pressure stimuli because they are more acceptable, gradually going over to lighter touch stimuli.

B. The Effect of Sensory Deficits

(1) Inhibition of motor functions
(2) Ignoral of the affected extremity
(3) Difficulty with coordination
(4) Difficulty with writing
(5) Danger of injury
(6) Dependence on visual control
(7) Delayed perception of sensory stimuli

Why do occupational therapists try to improve sensory deficits? To explain this, and also to plan an appropriate treatment programme, one has to look at the resulting disability occurring with sensory deficits.

(1) Inhibition of Motor Functions

Tactile-kinaesthetic disturbances can influence motor function considerably. Spontaneous recovery, as well as treatment success, depends on intact sensation. Patients with severe sensory loss have no inclination to move. Manipulation can become clumsy, uncoordinated and sometimes even ataxic. In order to differentiate between a sensory deficit and an apraxia, detailed testing is essential.

(2) Ignoral of the Affected Extremity

The non-use, neglect or total ignoral of the affected side may be explained as follows: Purposeful, controlled movements are normally guided and monitored through tactile-kinaesthetic modalities. The sensory feedback makes sure that the movement sequence is correct. A hand lacking these essential sensory qualities is not used automatically. If a patient constantly loses objects from his hand, knocks things over, or hits his limbs against furniture, he sees this as an accumulation of negative experiences and will stop using the arm altogether. As he has a second fully functional hand he will use it in preference to the affected one, even if it suffers no motor impairment.

(3) Difficulty with Coordination

The coordination and interplay between both hands is interrupted if the affected hand is not used spontaneously during practical activities. The sound hand is brought automatically and quickly towards the object, whereas the affected one is slow, hesitant and cannot help during manipulations.

(4) Difficulty with Writing

Even with good motor function, writing may be impaired if sensory deficits persist. Fluency is particularly affected, because this is possible only with diadochokinesis, which in turn is possible only with sensation.

(5) Danger of Injury

This is the most unpleasant effect. Burns, abrasions, cuts and bruises can occur if there is no sensation. The patient has to be especially careful during household activities or when returning to a manual job.

(6) Dependence on Visual Control

Without visual control a hand with severe sensory loss cannot carry out such activities as getting an object out of a pocket or handbag, tucking shirt or blouse into the back of trousers or skirts while dressing, or fastening a zip or tying an apron behind the back.

(7) Delayed Perception of Sensory Stimuli

Patients with brain injury frequently show a delayed perception of sensory stimuli although adequate sensation is present. During the temperature test, using two small tubes, one filled with hot water and one with cold water, for example, the patient cannot tell the difference if the stimuli are given in quick succession. If the stimuli are put onto the arm for a longer period of time, however, and the therapist allows a time lapse between the two, the patient can identify them correctly. The same reaction can be observed during the stereognosis test. The object is recognised only slowly and after a prolonged period of time.

Published work describing this delayed perception is scarce, but it is. possible that a delayed feedback within the areas of perception, integration and coordination is responsible. Perhaps these patients can perceive only a fraction of the stimulus that is then, with difficulty, put together as a whole.

Whatever the explanation for delayed perception of sensation, it explains why the affected hand is not used spontaneously even if reasonable motor and sensory functions are present. During treatment we have to consider these delayed reactions.

C. Testing Sensation

(1) Prerequisites
(2) Practical testing of sensation
(3) Observations
(4) Test material is not treatment material
(5) Reassessment for further treatment planning
(6) Elimination of visual and auditory control

Each hemiplegic patient should be tested for sensation at the beginning of rehabilitation, as well as at frequent intervals during therapy. For a detailed assessment, certain factors have to be present.

(1) Prerequisites

(a) Attention and cooperation
(b) Rapport and trust
(c) Intact motor functions
(d) Starting position
(e) Temperature of the hand

(f) Understanding the English language
(g) Testing both extremities
(h) Application of stimuli at irregular intervals
(i) Enough time and a peaceful environment

(a) Attention and Cooperation A certain degree of attention span and cooperation is the basis for any type of testing. If the patient tires quickly the testing should be spread over more than one treatment session. If the attention span of the patient is very short the therapist should choose a quiet room to avoid distraction.

(b) Rapport and Trust This is essential and can be facilitated by establishing eye contact while sitting opposite the patient.

(c) Intact Motor Function This is the basis for testing such things as stereognosis. Impairment of motor function makes it difficult to assess the results adequately. The posture and movements of the whole body influence sensation. A patient with severe paralysis of the hand, whether flaccid or spastic, has to be guided by the therapist. This means she has to place his hands around the object and move it. This can never be the same as when a patient actively manipulates the object himself. *It is therefore essential to remember that with severe motor disability, stereognosis cannot be tested adequately although touch and deep sensation can be tested.*

(d) Starting Position The patient is usually tested while seated at a table, and the position of trunk and arm have to be controlled during testing. Sometimes the inhibition of spasticity needs to be carried out before testing can begin.

Neither testing nor treatment should take place within abnormal postural or movement patterns. Abnormal tone influences sensation negatively — for example, if arm and hand are fixed in flexor spasticity the stimuli over the tensed muscle are not felt in the same way as over the relaxed one. If the hand closes loosely and at the same time touches an object this is very different from gripping an object with flexor spasticity.

(e) Temperature of the Hand Normal temperature of the hand is the basis for tactile recognition. Circulatory problems as well as winter weather conditions may be the reason for cold hands particularly in outpatients. Gentle rubbing or alternating warm and cold baths can help to normalise the temperature. Sometimes a cup of tea will suffice.

(f) Understanding the English Language The patient should have a certain understanding of language in order to respond to instructions during testing. The result with non-English-speaking people, or with aphasic patients, should be looked at with caution. Generally speaking, instructions should be short, clear and concise so that the patient can understand them. They should also be the same for each individual and the therapist should avoid questions where more than one answer is possible. One should ask, for example: 'What is this?' or 'What are you holding in your hand?' rather than 'Is this a bowl or a spoon?'.

(g) Testing Both Extremities Both sides of the body should be tested so that the unaffected side can be used as a control against which any deficits of the affected side can be established. The therapist may identify problems — for example, if an object is not recognised with either hand this is an indication of a disturbance in form perception.

(h) Application of Stimuli at Irregular Intervals Tactile stimuli should be given at irregular intervals to assess the reactions to them correctly.

(i) Enough Time and a Peaceful Environment These are necessary to assess sensation. There should be an interval between two tactile stimuli so that one is eliminated before the next one is presented.

(2) Practical Testing of Sensation

(a) Superficial sensation
(b) Temperature
(c) Pain sensation
(d) Deep sensation
(e) Weight differentiation
(f) Stereognosis
(g) Form perception
(h) Other tests

(a) Superficial Sensation The different types of superficial sensations are tested at different points in the arm and hand.

> *Pressure* is tested with the finger only; using the fingernail could cause pain and should be avoided.
> Perception of *light touch* can be tested with cotton wool.
> Different *touch sensations, both sharp and blunt,* are tested with an

open safety pin with the therapist touching the patient alternately with the point and the round end.

The perception of superficial sensation is tested only in this manner and the patient is asked only if, when and how he felt the stimulus. If, in addition he is asked where he felt it this would fall within the area of body scheme.

(b) Temperature To test temperature difference (and not pain sensation) during extreme heat or cold, four different glass tubes filled with water at 0°C, 20°C, 40°C, and 60°C are used. Patients who have inadequate temperature sensation but have intact pain sensation are unable to feel the difference between the four tubes. They find stimulation with 0°C and 60°C painful but are unable to say whether it is hot or cold.

(c) Pain Sensation This is an important safety factor against injury and the therapist should not confine her judgement to the results of the safety-pin test or the temperature test. Only pinching the skin in different areas will give an indication of how great the danger of injury is with severe loss of sensation.

(d) Deep Sensation Changes of movement and position are tested in: shoulder; elbow; wrist; and fingers.

Without visual control the patient should establish in which direction flexion and extension are carried out. The sequence of movements are chosen at random and the patient has to indicate whether he feels the movement upwards or downwards, or whether his joint is stretched or bent lightly or fully. The therapist holds the side of the arm very lightly. This is important because the pressure of the therapist's hands on the flexors or extensors could give additional information to the patient.

Abrupt and extreme flexion and extension should also be avoided because through the overstretching of muscles, tendons and the joint capsule, pain sensation could influence proprioception.

If imitation with the sound arm is demanded, proprioception is being tested as well as body scheme. If the result is negative, it is not possible to decide correctly where the deficit lies.

(e) Weight Differentiation Materials: Six closed containers of equal form and size filled with lead pellets or cotton wool with the following

weights — 30, 40, 60, 100, 150 and 300 gm. This test is carried out only if normal grip functions are present.

The therapist starts by asking the patient to differentiate between the minimal 30 gm and the maximal 300 gm and then gradually works through the others. Depending on the professions of the various patients, weight differences within the range of 10 gm can be recognised only by those who carry out fine manual tasks.

(f) *Stereognosis* For testing the above, objects from daily life which vary in size, form, surface and material are used — for example, scissors, nailbrush, rubber, coin, match, screw. The objects should be ones that can be easily manipulated. As mentioned, if manipulation is difficult through impaired motor function the result is not valid.

For testing a patient with aphasia, the therapist can compensate by having each object duplicated so that he can point to the one he recognises after identifying the other in his hand.

(g) *Form Perception* The tactile recognition of geometric shapes is additional to the stereognosis test, and demands the ability to recognise a shape.

(h) *Other Tests* With most patients the above described tests are sufficient. Only if the profession of a patient demands a higher quality of sensation should the therapist undertake other tests such as those used for graphesthesia, two-point discrimination, or discrimination of bilateral tactile stimuli. All these tests are described in neurology books.

(3) Observations

If different sensory deficits exist simultaneously, establishing the individual one can be difficult. Sometimes patients can compensate and this in turn may result in false assessment. As an occupational therapist one is not only interested in the end result but also in how the patient behaves during the testing sessions. Each test sheet should have a large section for recording observations.

An example would be that during testing for stereognosis a coin may not be recognised as such, but as hard and cold. To record this as a failure would be incorrect. The object is recognised by temperature and consistency, but not by shape and size. For treatment planning this means that one can use the intact sensation as a basis for training the other deficits. First of all, the therapist can use metal (cold) and wooden (warm) objects, and later on she can use objects varying in size and shape but made out of the same material.

Observations made outside the formal test are equally important and revealing — for example, the practical manipulation and behaviour of the patient.

(4) Test Material is not Treatment Material

Material used for testing sensation is principally not used for treatment because repetition of the test cannot then be correctly judged.

(5) Reassessment for Further Treatment Planning

In the course of rehabilitation it is necessary from time to time to repeat sensation testing, in order to establish the success of treatment and also to see whether it is necessary to modify the programme.

(6) Elimination of Visual and Auditory Control

In daily life we use the function of more than one sense simultaneously and combine them to create a whole picture. For testing, however, as the therapist wants to establish the deficits, it is necessary to eliminate information from other sense modalities, particularly vision and hearing.

The various ways of eliminating vision have advantages and disadvantages which have to be taken into consideration.

The patient can be asked to put his hand behind his back. This is an unusual position for tactile and kinaesthetic perception and manipulation, which is normally carried out in front of the body at waist or chest height.

Putting a cloth over the patient's eyes should be avoided, because this can make him feel insecure, and the rapport between patient and therapist may be hindered considerably. Through the insecurity of not knowing what is happening to him the patient may feel suspicious and sometimes become giddy. These negative influences impair the cooperation and performance of the patient.

Closing the eyes has a similarly negative effect.

By turning the head to one side the therapist can eliminate visual control but only if the patient can be trusted not to cheat.

A cloth placed directly over the patient's hand eliminates vision

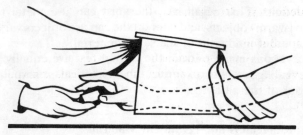

Figure 50. *Wooden construction with curtains used for stereognosis test.*

but also hinders the manipulation of objects. If, however, the patient selects objects out of a deep box, a towel over the top may be used. The patient is not hindered and visual control is eliminated.

If the patient is tested at a table a piece of cardboard can be held between his face and hands.

For testing and treatment, a stool-type wooden construction is useful. A large piece of cloth on the therapist's side and a curtain on the patient's side make it impossible to see the objects. Through the angle, the therapist is able to watch how the patient manipulates the objects (Fig 50).

A bag made from cloth (Fig 64) eliminates vision if the hand is placed inside and the patient is asked to feel for a particular object. This is the same as getting something out of a trouser pocket or a handbag.

To *eliminate auditory information*, a soft piece of cloth or felt can be put on the table. The patient is therefore unable to recognise an object by a particular noise. Some sounds are unavoidable such as that made when brushing the hand over an object.

D. Training Sensation

(1) Prerequisites of treatment
(2) Treatment planning (range)
(3) Practical treatment suggestions
(4) Treatment aims

The disabling effects of sensory deficits described above show why it is necessary to concentrate in occupational therapy on the treatment and improvement of sensory function. Nurses and physiotherapists should also bear in mind the effects of impaired sensation.

(1) Prerequisites of Treatment

(a) Normalising muscle tone
(b) Suitable working positions
(c) Stimulating sensation without increasing spasticity
(d) Cooperation of the patient
(e) Allowing sufficient time
(f) Consideration of other disabilities
(g) Repetition of stimuli
(h) Variation of stimuli
(i) Adjustment of training intensity

Occupational therapy treatment of motor function in the adult hemiplegic patient uses the Bobath method as its basis. Disturbance in tactile-kinaesthetic functions is also considered in other treatment methods. There is no special treatment method for sensory deficits designed for occupational therapy, although there are certain prerequisites that should be taken into account.

(a) Normalising Muscle Tone Severely altered muscle tone makes normal tactile-kinaesthetic functions impossible. Because of this the first and most important principles for sensation training are normalising muscle tone and eliminating abnormal postural and movement patterns.
The treatment of sensation cannot be separated from motor function and should always be considered as sensory-motor training.

(b) Suitable Working Positions The most suitable position for facilitating perception varies from patient to patient. Preferably, the patient should be allowed to work at waist or chest height. Sometimes, however, it is more suitable for the individual to work on a low stool or on the floor (Figs 58; 59).

(c) Stimulating Sensation without Increasing Spasticity Training sensation is always considered a stimulation therapy, particularly when facilitating touch sensatin but also when training proprioception. The therapist has to be trained in the various sensory stimulation techniques so that she does not increase spasticity through inappropriate stimuli. Hence, this has to be left to the experienced therapist.

(d) Cooperation of the Patient To achieve success in training sensation, as with any other training, the cooperation of the patient is necessary.

A certain concentration and alertness, as well as an understanding that the treatment is necessary, are all-important.

(e) Allowing Sufficient Time If it is established during testing that sensation is slowed down on the affected side, the therapist has to take this into consideration during treatment. If one is considering proprioception, then the patient is put into a reflex inhibiting position and kept there, so that he can feel what it is like before he is asked to move. The same procedure should be followed during tactile training, so that the patient has sufficient time to perceive the tactile stimuli correctly. The various materials should not be changed too quickly.

(f) Consideration of other Disabilities Hemianopia, aphasia, lack of spatial awareness and deficits in visual form perception should be considered in training sensation and should not be separated.

(g) Repetition of Stimuli The hemiplegic patient cannot usually recognise a sensory stimulus if it is given only once or twice. Repetition is therefore essential if he is to be able to perceive sensation correctly. The stimuli have to be repeated with each treatment session, every day and every week for as long as necessary — as with any other learning process.

Training proprioception means that the patient carries out movements not once or twice, but a hundred times until the proprioceptors of muscles, tendons and joints sense the movement again.

It has been found that adult hemiplegic patients in the final stages of recovery often show more deficits in sensation in the upper limbs than in their lower limbs. This is mainly due to the leg being used for standing and walking, which in itself is a sensory stimulus. The arm, however, does not receive this stimulus automatically in daily life; therefore it is essential that intensive training of sensation start as early as possible.

(h) Variation of Stimuli It is important that the patient receive a variety of tactile-kinaesthetic experiences, because this is what occurs in our normal environment. The selection should contain different elements such as pieces of games made from different materials (Fig 63), and variation of movement sequences through the positioning of the pieces in different directions.

(i) Adjustment of Training Intensity The tactile activities should be planned according to the abilities of the patient. The level of an activity can be too high, and the therapist can demand too much of a patient.

This can have a negative effect — for example, if a patient with severe astereognosis is asked to find small objects from a box filled with sand. The various grades of difficulties are described as follows.

(2) Treatment Planning (Range)

(a) Combined perception of different sense modalities with the possibility of compensating	— Tactile-kinaesthetic perception only, without the possibility of compensating
(b) Gross discrimination	— Detailed discrimination
(c) To estimate	— To be exact
(d) Large differences	— Small differences
(e) Three-dimensional	— Two-dimensional
(f) To pick up single objects placed by the therapist	— To pick up single objects from a large number

The test results are the foundation for planning and grading treatment. The therapist has to consider whether loss of sensation is specific or general. The treatment of sensation is not achieved by presenting any material at random but only through the selection of the appropriate stimuli. Treatment is graded from easy activities to more advanced ones.

(a) Combined perception of different sense modalities with the possibility of compensating — Tactile-kinaesthetic perception only, without the possibility of compensating To make tactile-kinaesthetic perception possible the therapist uses other senses at the beginning. The different senses are closely interlinked and complement each other. Only rarely is just one sense connected with a particular perception process.

A normal, non-injured person rarely uses his tactile functions in isolation. What he can feel, he can also see, smell or hear. It is often not enough to go into a shop and look at an item like fruit or fabric, but also to touch and perhaps taste it. Sometimes sense of smell also helps in the choice of an item. At other times, the merchandise may be rubbed or tapped to test quality.

If a non-injured person uses such a variety of sense impressions a patient certainly needs them as well. Only the simultaneous perception of different sensations make correct information possible. That is why, at the beginning of treatment, visual control and any other chance of compensating are not eliminated.

Examples

In the first stages of training the patient is allowed to see and hear the object that he feels. In the second stage a piece of cardboard is held above the hands. In the third stage a thick cloth is put on the table to eliminate sound, so that pure tactile-kinaesthetic recognition is demanded.

A patient with astereognosis may be able to differentiate between temperature and weight. Using this as a basis the therapist firstly practises with heavy and light as well as cold and warm objects (metal, wood, textiles). During the course of treatment, compensation is eliminated by presenting different objects made from the same material.

Such gradings can sometimes be presented in one treatment session — for example, the patient is allowed to manipulate objects with visual control, use the objects as a game, and afterwards he may hide them in a box of sand. Only when these objects have been recognised in a tactile and visual sense can the patient be asked to differentiate between them on a tactile-kinaesthetic level.

(b) Gross Discrimination — Detailed Discrimination It is necessary to remember that it is easier to discriminate between objects that are totally different than between those with little difference.

Firstly, the patient is allowed to sort objects according to *one* quality — for example, sorting according to weight, size, consistency, shape or texture. In practice, this may mean all roughly textured objects at the right and all smooth ones at the left; or, out of a collection, round objects are selected first and then square ones. Only later on is the patient asked to select a small square object and a large round one out of a collection of various shapes and sizes.

(c) To Estimate — To Be Exact The patient is now asked to estimate the quantity through touch — whether there are a few or many marbles in a box. To upgrade the task the patient is asked to establish the exact number of marbles. It is easier if there are only marbles in the container and more difficult if they are placed among other things, which would mean that they had to be picked out individually and counted.

(d) Large Differences — Small Differences
Example
From a box filled with grit or sand the patient has to find, firstly, large objects then, secondly, smaller ones. The differences between object and grit or sand become smaller and smaller, and increase in difficulty.

(e) Three-Dimensional — Two-Dimensional In general, it is easier to recognise through touch three-dimensional objects like dice, balls, cylinders or pyramids, than two-dimensional circles, squares, rectangles or triangles cut out of thin cardboard. It is also easier to feel for a key, spoon or a clothes peg than to establish them on a tactile basis when made out of cardboard.

(f) To pick up single objects placed by the therapist — To pick up single objects from a large number A relatively easy task is demanded of the patient if the therapist puts an object in his hand and he has to recognise it through touch. It is considerably more difficult to select a clothes peg or half a candle from several other objects.

(3) Practical Treatment Suggestions

As already mentioned, treatment must be adjusted to the individual's needs. Only three main points are mentioned here as treatment suggestions.
   (a) Training sensation when there is severe motor disability
   (b) Facilitation of sensory-motor functions with mainly proprioceptive deficits
   (c) Training sensation when there are deficits in touch sensation
   A strict separation of treatment suggestions with disturbed proprioception and touch sensation is impossible, because both sense modalities are closely linked. Normal activities of daily living demand both qualities at the same time. That is why the described treatment suggestions aim at facilitating sensation as a whole, sometimes with more emphasis on proprioception, sometimes more on light sensation. The treatment of astereognosis needs the stimulation of both areas.

(a) Training Sensation when there is Severe Motor Disability During the first stage of rehabilitation of an adult hemiplegic patient, the emphasis is often on improving motor functions, but stimulation of tactile-kinaesthetic functions can be incorporated at the same time as motor and sensory functions and they should not be separated.

Using one of the board games bilaterally, as shown in Figs 26 and 27, the patient is asked to grasp the pegs, which are covered with different materials thereby facilitating sensation (Fig 51).

Thick cylinders (diameter about 5 cm) covered with round headed nails, sandpaper, leather, foam, wire, rope or other kinds of materials, may also enhance tactile perception (Figs 23; 24; 52).

By pushing hands along the top of the table, as in a matching game

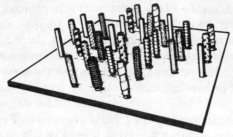

Figure 51. *Solitaire rods covered with different materials.*

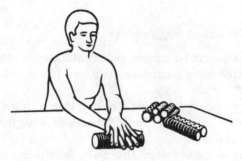

Figure 52. *Bilateral rolling of large rods which are covered with different materials.*

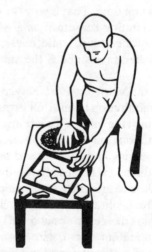

Figure 53. *Weightbearing on different surfaces for tactile-kinaesthetic stimulation.*

shown in Fig 31, tactile stimulation is achieved through friction.

Weightbearing through the affected arm (Figs 11a; 11b; 39; 40) facilitates motor function as well as proprioception. Reciprocal innervation is necessary to stabilise the arm, and thus promote proprioceptive perception of this particular position. At the same time, muscle tone is normalised and associated reactions are avoided.

Touch sensation in the hand can also be facilitated by using different surfaces for weightbearing — for example, wood or metal surfaces, foam, towelling, carpet squares, sand or pebbles. These stimuli can be pleasant or sometimes unpleasant for the patient (Fig 53). Through the change in the weightbearing surface the hand receives different pressure sensations and therefore a multitude of stimuli are given to the neglected arm.

As the patient improves in motor as well as sensation functions, the therapist can start using bimanual techniques, whereby the weightbearing hand is used to stabilise different objects like a wooden board or a cane mat (Fig 53).

(b) Facilitation of Sensory Motor Functions with mainly Proprioceptive Deficits During functional training proprioception cannot be separated from movement. If severe loss is present the therapist usually guides the movements of the patient to re-establish a feeling for them. The next step could be that the patient himself controls the movement of his affected arm with his sound one. Bilateral activities are indicated at this stage (see Chapter V).

As an upgrading, the movements of the affected arm are only indirectly guided with the sound arm. This means bimanual activities are carried out — for example, lifting large objects as in Fig 41. In order for the proprioceptors of muscles, tendons and joints to receive a variety of stimulation and information, bimanual and unilateral activities are varied in direction and strength.

If grip function is possible, different remedial games may be played where the pieces have to be grasped from different directions (up, down, left, right, back, in front). In order to use the right amount of strength the patient is asked to manipulate light as well as heavier objects. Movements against resistance give similar stimuli to the proprioceptor, as is the case when weightbearing, but here it is linked with movement. During sanding (upwards, horizontal, downwards) the different grades of sandpaper and the hardness of the wood provide the resistance. Patients who cannot control their movements, and sometimes even have ataxic movements as a result of a deficit in proprioception, become more competent at controlling and guiding their movements through this type of resistance.

As a next step in the treatment plan, fine skilled movements without any resistance must be practised.

It is difficult to improve diadochokinesis even with near intact motor functions. Clapping hands facilitates diadochokinesis as well as co-ordination. Patient and therapist sit opposite each other. First of all, both clap their hands on their thighs, then the palms are clapped together. For this the forearms have to turn. The next step could be to clap each other's hands. Here the patient has such additional controls as visual and auditory through the clapping, and tactile through contact with his own hands or the therapist's hands.

During ADL training a hemiplegic patient who lacks proprioception may have considerable difficulties — for example, while dressing, the hand may stay in the sleeve because the patient does not have the feel for extension in his elbow. Manipulations behind the back where no visual control of the movement is possible, like fastening a garment are particularly difficult. Here only tactile-kinaesthetic functions can be used.

The therapist can practise the movement by passing objects through a tube, or by passing different objects from one hand to the other in different shoulder and elbow positions. The patient is successful doing this in front and next to his body where visual control is still guaranteed. The changeover above the head or behind the back or neck is considerably more difficult. Such increase from light to more difficult activities in the treatment plan will eventually lead to the treatment goal — for example, the patient can tuck his shirt into his trousers, fasten a back zip, or tie an apron behind the back.

There are some activities that need distance perception — for example, if a patient is sweeping with a very long handled broom or weaving, where the movement and the visual control are spatially quite distant from each other and are achieved through proprioception. Other examples are watering flowers and pouring coffee. Such activities are very difficult for patients lacking proprioception and can be incorporated into treatment only later.

If the patient needs to practise proprioception in his fingers he may be asked to grasp different-sized objects, where his hand has to close sometimes tightly, sometimes more widely. The game described in Fig 54 is particularly good because differently-sized discs are used.

To train proprioception distally the therapist can, on the one hand, choose activities that give pressure to the inside of the hand as is the case when grasping hard objects or, on the other hand, she should use activities that do the same thing to the outside of the fingers; something

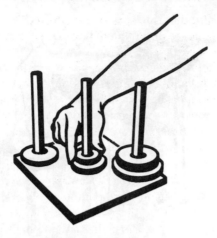

Figure 54. *Span game with wooden discs.*

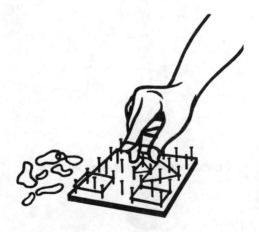

Figure 55. *Making patterns with rubber band on a pinboard.*

that is achieved by using rubber bands spread over a pinboard making geometric patterns (Fig 55).

Macrame also uses flexion and extension of the fingers, and needs fine skilled movements and proprioception. These activities are carried out only with patients who have negligible deficits to start with, or those who have made good recovery during treatment.

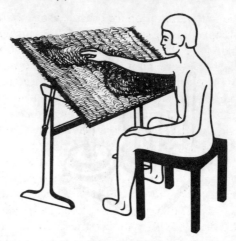

Figure 56. *Stroking a piece of carpet with the palm.*

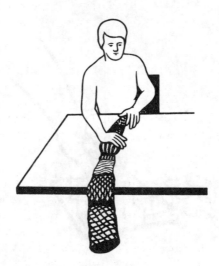

Figure 57. *Pushing round objects through a tube made of different fabrics.*

(c) Training Sensation when there are Deficits in Touch Sensation In the last part of the treatment suggestions the emphasis will be on the disturbances of touch sensation.

To begin with these stimuli have to be administered quite strongly if the patient is to feel them at all. The various stimuli are tapping, rubbing and brushing and are carried out at the beginning of each treatment session, in preparation for other sensory training for manual activities. Washing, applying soap, rinsing and drying with a towel, and rubbing cream on have the same effect and may be done either by the therapist or by the patient himself. Even so, care must be taken to ensure that one does not increase spasticity through these sensory stimuli. The therapist has to watch posture and movements as well as the quality of muscle tone after each stimulation. If the patient has severe spasticity such stimulation should perhaps be avoided altogether, because it may do more harm than good.

During tactile stimulation the therapist can either keep the arm and hand still while an object passes over them, or the patient may move his hand over the object, combining tactile with kinaesthetic input. Pieces of carpet with different pile may be fixed to a vertical surface and the patient asked to draw shapes with his affected hand. If he moves his hand in the opposite direction the drawing is rubbed out (Fig 56).

Other types of stimulation

Drawing patterns on a table surface. If the hand does not move easily talcum powder or soap and water make it easier.

Rubbing out on a blackboard with the palm. Through friction an intensive tactile stimulation is created.

The tube shown in Fig 57 is made up out of different fabrics. By extending arm and hand, small balls (less resistance) or bigger ones (increased resistance) are pushed through it. Here the hand receives different tactile sensations varying from section to section.

This polishing, rubbing or stroking is also necessary for everyday activities like folding linen or paper, or when making a bed and smoothing the sheets.

Pulses are used in occupational therapy in different ways. Activities can be varied by using larger ones (beans, peas, corn) or medium (lentils, millet, rice) or the very fine-sized grains (cornmeal, sugar, flour). Gravel and sand are also suitable for sensation training. If put into a container the patient can burrow his hands into them, push them from one corner to the other or make patterns.

Depending on the stage of treatment, objects varying in size and shape are hidden and the patient is asked to feel for them among the different materials.

The positioning of the activity is most important because abnormal posture and movement patterns impair tactile sensation. It might, for example, be too difficult for the patient to carry out this activity at waist height because he could use his arm in shoulder retraction, internal rotation, elbow flexion, pronation and flexion of the wrist. In this case, the correct positioning of the bowl is on a low stool or on the

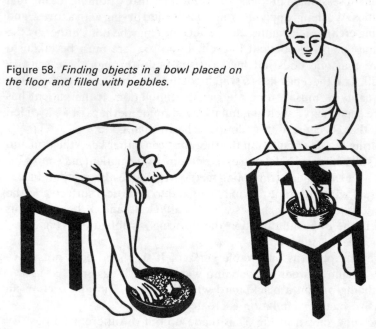

Figure 58. *Finding objects in a bowl placed on the floor and filled with pebbles.*

Figure 59. *Finding objects hidden in rice with vision excluded. The bowl is positioned on a low stool.*

floor, in order to inhibit abnormal movements and facilitate normal ones, thus improving sensation (Figs 58; 59).

Using wooden or cardboard objects, shown in Fig 59, ensures that the patient uses only tactile-kinaesthetic information to find the hidden objects.

Firstly, the patient is asked to pick out all the objects, then to name them as he picks them out; the third step will be to find a specific object that is buried in the cornmeal (Fig 60). This activity can also be used with aphasic patients by having a second set of the objects that are in the container out on a tray and asking the patient to point to them. The wooden frame with a piece of cloth eliminates vision (Figs 50;60).

Figure 61 shows another possible way of promoting tactile sensation. The coarse and fine materials are kept in the hand, then released in a constant flow to make patterns on the table surface. Afterwards these patterns are eliminated by moving the palm over them (Fig 62). A big box of sand is a useful piece of equipment for making such patterns.

Figure 52 shows how big cylinders covered with different materials

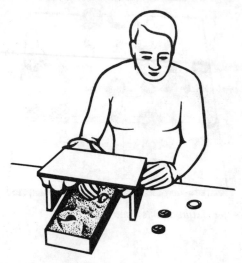

Figure 60. *Searching for a particular object hidden in cornflour, at table height.*

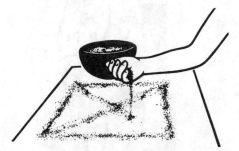

Figure 61. *Making patterns on a table with sand; hand semi-closed.*

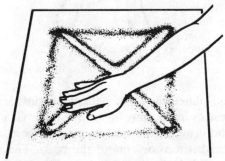

Figure 62. *Making patterns on a table with sand; hand open.*

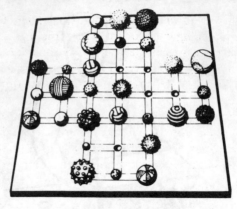

Figure 63. *Differently textured balls used as pieces of a game.*

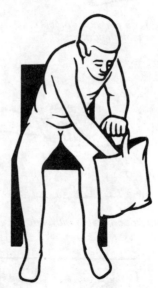

Figure 64. *Finding an object in a bag with affected arm in spasticity inhibiting position.*

are manipulated bilaterally. If the patient has sufficient hand function at this stage these cylinders may be used unilaterally in different ways: rolling in pronation and supination, or passing them from one hand to the other, either in front or behind the body. The more varied the surfaces of these cylinders, the more varied the tactile stimulation for the patient. If the therapist makes pairs of each cylinder she can put one into the patient's sound hand and with the affected one the patient must find the matching cylinder from the others.

The solitaire game is particularly useful because it requires frequent grip and grip-release of the pieces. This advantage is incorporated into the training of sensation by covering the pegs with different materials (Fig 51).

Figure 63 shows a variation. Here different balls made out of metal, wood, cork, rubber, wool or polystyrene are used and also ping-pong balls and pine cones. These different balls give uneven tactile and proprioceptive information depending on their weight, size and material.

If the individual pieces are picked out of an open box, the patient can use his eyes as well. Nevertheless, it is much more difficult if the objects have to be selected out of a bag without visual control. Again, positioning of box and bag is most important for preventing abnormal patterns. One possibility is to let the bag hang between the patient's legs. Another is to hold it with the unaffected hand on the unaffected side, so that the affected arm has to cross midline facilitating shoulder protraction, normal tone and tactile sensations.

The surfaces of the dice shown in Fig 65 are covered with different materials. Nails with rounded heads, metal, leather, fur or sandpaper. Again, these are made in duplicate. The patient has one in either hand and is asked to turn the same surface to the top. Depending on the stage of treatment different pairs are given, covered either with coarser or finer materials. Dice with numbers indicated either with holes or round headed nails may also be matched.

To facilitate coordination at this stage, the therapist can cover the hoop shown in Fig 48 with a sisal cord to stimulate the hand. A rope made out of different strings and cords, a tube made out of different fabrics (Fig 57), as well as material remnants that are knotted together, may be used for these activities. To facilitate not only tactile but also kinaesthetic input the therapist varies the position of the materials. Sometimes the patient is asked to grip from up to down or vice versa, but also horizontally and diagonally.

If the patient has good motor function the therapist can use a technique that facilitates coordination of both hands as well as sensation. Figure 66 shows weaving with a rough sisal cord, but the affected hand is often not used spontaneously in this process. To give the affected hand an equal chance the glove is put on the sound hand. *If the over-activity of the sound hand is inhibited the functions in the affected one are facilitated.*

Many activities may be used and examples include: pottery; collages

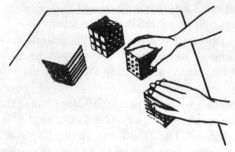

Figure 65. *Dice covered with different materials used for training superficial sensation.*

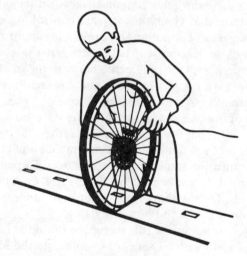

Figure 66. *Round weaving with a glove on the sound hand.*

made out of different papers screwed into little balls; polishing activities; washing small garments by hand; kneading dough and forming into shapes (balls, rolls, brezel and other shapes); and mixing minced meat and forming it into meatballs.

(4) Treatment Aims

   (a) To prevent injury
   (b) Compensation
   (c) To promote tactile discrimination
   (d) Well coordinated movements

(e) Spontaneous use of the affected hand
(f) Coordination of both hands
(g) To give the patient a feeling of success
(h) Discharge

During all forms of treatment the therapist has certain short-term and long-term aims for each individual patient. This also applies to the training of sensation.

(a) To Prevent Injury Preventing injury is an important aim and it has to be minimised if not completely prevented. The patient needs to compensate, particularly during household activities and work assessments. With certain professions work habits need to be changed — for example, the patient should hold an onion with the sound hand and use the knife in the affected one but this is possible only if he has good

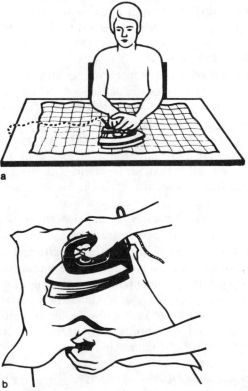

Figures 67a and 67b. *(a) Bilateral ironing (with guard). (b) Unilateral ironing (with guard).*

motor function. In addition, adaptations can prevent injury. An iron may be fitted with a guard so that burns are prevented if the hand loses its grip. If a severe disability persists the iron may safely be used bilaterally (Fig 67a).

If arm and hand functions are present but sensory deficits persist, the affected hand holds the iron and the sound one performs the more dangerous functions like holding or smoothing the garment near the tip of the iron (Fig 67b).

(b) Compensation As with all disabilities the therapist has to ask the following questions with sensory deficits: 'How far can the deficit be retrained and improved?' 'Is compensation necessary?' 'Does compensation training prevent the improvement which could be achieved through specific treatment?'

During testing all possibilities of compensation have to be eliminated as the actual deficit needs to be established. Sometimes during treatment, however, one cannot do without compensation.

Compensation in the motor area when practising functional activities should always be avoided. In the area of sensation, however, the therapist has to look critically at whether the patient might not be harmed if he is not given the chance to compensate. Many patients find their own ways of compensating, particularly when long-term sensory deficits exist. If, however, a patient does not find these for himself the therapist can suggest the following to him.

Visual compensation is one of the most important ways of compensating. This is even more important for a patient with a combined sensory-motor disability than for a patient who has 'only' motor deficits. Only if the hand is forward within the visual field is control over it guaranteed.

Tactile control can be carried out with the sound hand — for example, when testing the temperature of the water that comes out of a tap the sound hand is used first before the affected one is washed.

Auditory control is a third possibility. The patient can discriminate through hearing whether a container is full or empty.

By compensating for the tactile-kinaesthetic sense, using other senses, the use of the affected extremity should be made possible. The aim of treatment is not the improvement of the test result but the best possible rehabilitation of the individual patient.

(c) To Promote Tactile Discrimination If possible, the therapist should try to achieve aims other than compensation. Through stimuli that facilitate sensation she wants to improve the patient's ability to discri-

minate between various tactile sensations, which give him better information about his environment.

(d) Well Coordinated Movements Through improvement of proprioception the therapist wants to achieve controlled movements that are not carried out consciously but automatically.

(e) Spontaneous Use of the Affected Hand Through lack of tactile-kinaesthetic information the patient does not receive enough motor impulses, and this may lead to the neglect of the affected side. It is an important treatment aim that the patient learns to bring his hand and arm into the visual field, and let it participate in the activity. The long-term aim is the spontaneous use of his hand.

(f) Coordination of Both Hands Combined with the training of the automatic and spontaneous use of the hand is the good coordination of both hands.

(g) To Give the Patient a Feeling of Success The desired treatment aims are only achieved if the demands put on the patient are adjusted to the stage reached in his rehabilitation. Success may be achieved if treatment is graded so that the patient can only just fulfil the task. Through this he will get a positive feedback.

(h) Discharge The therapist has to ask herself how much time is necessary to achieve the optimum improvement in the patient's condition, with regard to sensory deficits — as with motor disturbances. A few days training, sometimes a few weeks, is not enough to improve effectively the severe sensation disturbances of an adult brain-injured patient. Sometimes a newly injured patient needs to be treated for several months. Some cases show improvement after one or two years. If improvement reaches a plateau over a longer period of time, despite intensive therapy, the therapist should decide whether continuing treatment is justified.

The profession of a patient should be taken into consideration when setting long-term treatment aims.

(5) Final Remarks

The disturbances in sensation with their tests and treatment methods have been described in detail in this chapter. This is important in the treatment of hemiplegia because sensory functions cannot be separated from motor functions.

The therapist has to look for abnormal postural and movement patterns because they influence tactile and proprioceptive functions considerably. Positions and movements that are carried out in reflex inhibiting positions with normal muscle tone receive more normal proprioceptive information than spastic muscles. If the arm is internally rotated, flexed and pronated with spasticity, tactile sensation may be different from when the arm is in external rotation, extended and supinated. Only the combination of controlled movements, as well as superficial and deep sensation, can lead to tactile-kinaesthetic recognition.

During treatment the first priority, if at all possible, is regaining and improving sensation, compensation being only a secondary priority. The treatment aim in occupational therapy is achieved when the patient is able to use his affected side as normally as possible in his activities of daily living. Even if for some reason this is not achieved with every patient, one should try all the various methods and use the ability of the central nervous system to relearn.

The practical observations are as follows. If a total disturbance of sensation persists and all stimuli have no effect, continuing treatment would be a waste of time. Even so, if only minimal deficits exist I suggest that treatment should always be continued.

During the acute phase, spontaneous recovery is sometimes improved and speeded up.

Finally, the facilitation of partially existent sensation is always worth while, even if only minimal improvement is achieved. If the lost functions are not regained they can be compensated for by the improvement of existing ones.

In order to be successful with treatment one always has to combine sensation with motor training. Through the correct choice of inhibition, facilitation and stimulation the therapist achieves an improvement in the quality of movement functions.

VIII Controlled One-Handed Training

A. During 'maintenance therapy'
B. With apraxia
C. During activities of daily living
D. During writing practice
E. During work rehabilitation (including household training)

Even if the emphasis of treatment is on the deficits and disturbances of the hemiplegic side, the therapist cannot ignore or even suppress activity on the sound side.

If normal function of the arm or hand is lost through amputation, peripheral or cerebral lesions, in principle it is necessary to promote dexterity in the sound hand, particularly if the dominant one is affected. Such dexterity training should not take place by excluding the paralysed extremity, which should be used for holding and supporting functions. If, for example, a severe disability is present the affected arm can hold the paper while the sound hand writes.

Under no circumstances should isolated one-handed training take place in occupational therapy. All activities of daily living should be carried out with consideration and incorporation of the affected side. If this is not done, asymmetric posture, spine deformities, contractures and pain may result. These can be avoided through bilateral and bimanual activities as well as through good control of the hemiplegic side during one-handed training.

These controls are as follows
Symmetrical trunk posture during sitting and standing;
Controlled posture or positioning of the paralysed arm and leg;
Avoidance of associated reactions in the affected arm and leg;

Avoidance of injuries and bedsores, particularly when sensory deficits are present;

Constant visual control of the affected side, even during unilateral activities with the sound hand;

The best possible incorporation of the paralysed side through holding and supporting functions during activities; and

Facilitation of coordination through bilateral and bimanual activities, even if the sound side is more active.

Only if these points are all considered can one-handed training be called 'controlled'.

A. Controlled One-Handed Training During Maintenance Therapy

This kind of treatment is indicated with older and severely disabled patients in long-term geriatric wards or homes. The activities, which are mainly carried out in groups, are limited to one-handed exercises.

Even if no functional improvement is expected with some long-standing hemiplegic patients, the danger of increased spasticity, contractures, asymmetrical posture, back pain and other pain, still exists. That is why during any activities with the sound hand the affected side needs good positioning (see Chapter V — Stage 1). It is equally important to avoid associated reactions (see Chapter III — 3b.).

B. Controlled One-Handed Training with Apraxia

Depending on the site of the lesion in the central nervous system, a hemiplegic patient may also have an apraxia. Without going into the details of the different forms of apraxia, it is obvious that it is an additional handicap and can depress the patient immensely. While the function of one hand is impaired through the hemiplegia, the other one, too, may be unable to function adequately because of apraxia. Patients are frustrated by not being able to eat, use scissors, put their glasses on for reading or being unable to fold them and put them into their case.

With such bilateral, but different, disabilities the therapist positions the hemiplegic arm correctly and then concentrates on the improvement of the apraxic side, using appropriate activities. Often the patient is helped by the therapist who guides the movement of the apraxic hand during manipulations. By doing this the patient is helped to get the feeling for different movement sequences.

Although little is known about the prognosis and the specific treatment of apraxia, the therapist should always try to experiment with different techniques.

C. Controlled One-Handed Training During Activities of Daily Living

Functional training and the training of activities of daily living in the treatment of hemiplegia should not be separated in occupational therapy but should be used in combination. Body symmetry, arm positioning, avoidance of associated reactions and abnormal patterns, as well as an improvement in the functional quality on the hemiplegic side, are prepared for by functional training and should be carried over into all activities of daily living.

Some Activities of Daily Living
   Independent eating, including cutting meat and buttering a slice of
   bread;
   Independent dressing;
   Personal hygiene, including shaving, manicure, using make-up,
   bathing or showering;
   Mobility, e.g. independent wheelchair mobility without causing
   associated reactions;
   Practical activities like making a telephone call, using money and
   shopping.

As most of the techniques and different ways of practising activities of daily living are known to most occupational therapists, only a few additional ones for controlled one-handed training during dressing are given.

Instruction in one-handed undressing and dressing is needed by most hemiplegic patients because most will not regain complete function in the arm and hand. In this area, occupational therapists have to work closely with nurses and physiotherapists and pass information regarding the stage of treatment reached to the other professions.

Bases for Starting Dressing
   Motivation of the patient

Time and quiet
Adequate sitting balance
Consideration of sensory deficits
Compensation abilities with hemianopia
Establishing body scheme disorders (dressing apraxias)
Establishing the neglect of the affected side
Establishing deficits in spatial relations (perception of garments in relation to the body)
Ability to understand, even without verbal communication, through imitation

In order not to demand too much or frustrate the hemiplegic patient with ADL training, the therapist should make sure that he fulfils these prerequisites; otherwise, she has to prepare these individually.

To give the patient the necessary security he should not sit on a high bed during dressing practice but on a normal chair. If the patient is frightened, another chair may be put at either side (Fig 69). The therapist sits in front but mostly towards the affected side of the patient. During washing and dressing in the early stages, the patient should take partial responsibility for his affected side. This is increased during later stages until he can fully incorporate his affected side.

Some Practical Examples. While the nurse still washes the patient, he should be encouraged at least to wash face, neck and chest and his affected arm. This is important for the integration of the hemiplegic side and body scheme. During this process the patient himself — and not the nurse — puts his affected arm into the sink. Later the patient also has to wash his sound arm and back for himself.

If the hemiplegic patient is dressed by the nurse he must himself put his affected arm into the sleeve.

At a later stage, when the patient can dress his top half independently, Figs 68a and 68b show how this is possible without elbow flexion, shoulder retraction and rotation in the body axis. The sleeve hangs between both legs and the arm is put forwards and downwards into it (Fig 68a).

While the garment is put onto the shoulder, the patient still leans forwards and the affected arm stays between his legs (Fig 68b). This position inhibits retraction of the shoulder and elbow flexion.

To put on or take off shoes, socks, stockings and trousers, crossing the legs is necessary and desirable because this facilitates sitting balance at the same time. If lifting the hemiplegic leg is not possible in a controlled manner, clasped hands are used to achieve this (Fig 69).

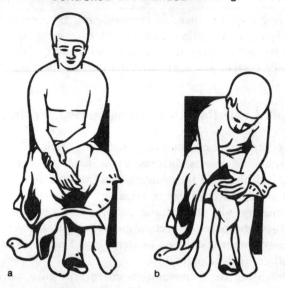

Figures 68a and 68b. *(a) Positioning of sleeve for inserting affected arm. (b) Leaning forwards during the dressing process.*

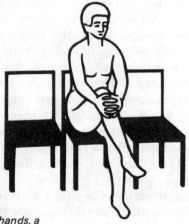

Figure 69. *Crossing legs using clasped hands, a chair on either side gives security to the patient.*

In contrast with other physical disabilities, early independence with a hemiplegic patient should not be achieved at all costs. The dangers of uncontrolled one-handed training are too great for this.

Activities of daily living are always carried out in the early stages with the help of the therapist. Only in the later stages will the patient take control himself.

By avoiding pure one-handed training, and by incorporating the hemiplegic side in the various activities, the training of activities of daily living becomes a part of the functional training. With increased independence it will once again become part of the patient's life.

D. Controlled One-Handed Training During Writing Practice

While concentrating on motor dysfunctions, deficits in sensation, apraxia, visual field defects, disturbances of form perception and construction, it is difficult for the occupational therapist to decide at what point, if at all, to start writing practice.

Before starting with an aphasic patient, she should consult the speech therapist because the occupational therapist is concerned only with the sensory-motor abilities of writing and not with the specific problems of an aphasic patient.

While practising these movements correct posture, correct table height, adequate lighting, correct positioning of the pad and the holding of the pen are essential.

If the paralysis of the dominant hand is irreversible practice should be started with the non-dominant one. As with all other one-handed activities, the hemiplegic arm should not be under the table but should hold the paper. If for some reason an object is used to hold the paper, the affected arm should be correctly positioned on the table, i.e. forearm inclusive of elbow and hand are next to the paper. A suitable positioning of the arm during one-handed typing is shown in Fig 21.

If the dominant side is only lightly disabled, or there is spontaneous recovery, writing may be practised by using an adaptation on the pen — for example, an enlarged grip. Depending on the patient the therapist decides on either a pencil, pen, felt-tip pen, chalk or fountain pen, as well as a hard, soft, thick or thin pen.

Suggestions for Carrying Out Writing Training. As a preparation, activities are chosen that facilitate the movement sequences of writing. On the one hand, these are loose fluent movements of shoulder girdle and upper arm to move hand and forearm along. On the other hand, they consist of quick alternating movements of wrist and fingers necessary for guiding the pen. These movements may be practised during, for example, ironing, polishing a table, or erasing a blackboard, painting with hands or a thick brush, painting big surfaces like murals, and also by using a thin brush to wax paper or fabric during batik.

In the early stage the patient can practise on a table surface or a blackboard as paper is likely to tear because the patient cannot control the pen adequately.

Grading Fluent Writing Ability. To begin with, big round forms are practised and these are repeated until they become fluent (1). These are big circles, spirals, ovals in every horizontal or diagonal position, figures of eight horizontally or vertically. Such big movements may be used later on to relax the affected arm. This is particularly important when practising the small and more complex movements which can tire the patient easily. One can also practise without a pen using the palm to follow a form on a blackboard until it is no longer visible. Below are some examples of movement directions that should be repeated again and again.

As a next step the size may be varied (2). Then the form or direction are changed but similar movements are used (3). At a later stage continuous forms are chosen with constant change in direction. Before practising words, letters are combined (4). Only after this, are words practised.

The therapist looks at the fluency of the movements rather than the neatness of the writing, because the effort of writing neatly may cause cramps and could easily tire the patient. Only gradually is he asked to write smaller, in normal size, between lines and, in addition to the round shape, introduce more and more straight and square shapes.

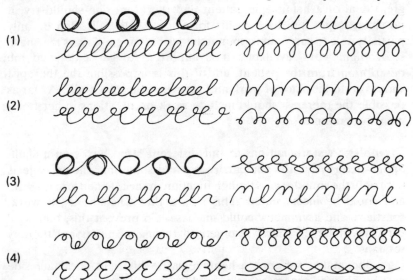

During this training, the therapist should establish the extent to which the patient uses writing professionally or privately. Is it very important to him? Given the complexity and the variety of movements during writing, it is hardly surprising if the patient does not achieve his former style, either in fluency or speed. After a hemiplegia one should be satisfied if the patient achieves a fairly legible, fluent handwriting.

E. Controlled One-Handed Training During Work Rehabilitation and During Household Activities

In the earlier treatment stages medical rehabilitation of the hemiplegic patient has priority; later, resettlement into the patient's own environment and possibly his return to work become more important.

After the initial intensive treatment period where motor, sensation and perceptive function have all been more or less successfully achieved the therapist has to decide whether these are adequate for a return to work. Unfortunately, a high proportion of adult brain-injured patients never regain the same amount of function in the arm and hand as in the leg, so that activities in the home or at work are carried out mainly by using the sound hand.

For resettlement back to work various different professions or trades have to be considered. Training for a different job demands a great deal of a hemiplegic patient and therefore one should try, if possible, to get him back to his former job. He will often be only partially able to carry out former activities but his employers may have some 'light work' available. It is important to get a detailed job description from the patient, and if this is impossible the therapist should go to his place of work and see what the job entails. As far as possible the therapist should include work preparations in her treatment programme.

Examples. A storeman has to put different sized boxes on a shelf. Spontaneously he lifts and carries big and sometimes heavy objects with only the sound arm, although function in the affected arm is useful and could be incorporated. This means that when he starts work, spasticity and asymmetry could increase. To prevent this, bimanual carrying of large objects is practised during occupational therapy sessions.

A clockmaker suffering a hemiplegia on his right dominant side made such good progress that he could carry out certain skilled movements with his affected hand. He used to work in a factory overseeing

15 workers and showing them the individual work processes; he also controlled the assembled watches before they were dispatched. His residual disability consisted of hemianopia, aphasia and perseveration. Resettlement to his former factory was possible but he was unable to carry out his former duties. As a preparation for the fine skilled movements that are necessary when assembling watches, he was asked in occupational therapy to pick up and sort small objects with a pair of tweezers and a pen-like instrument. Later, he made mosaics in the same way. Through this work simulation, the watchmaker learned to manipulate with his left hand the tweezers that he formerly held in his right hand. The fine handle of the other instrument had to be made longer and thicker so that the affected hand could grip it.

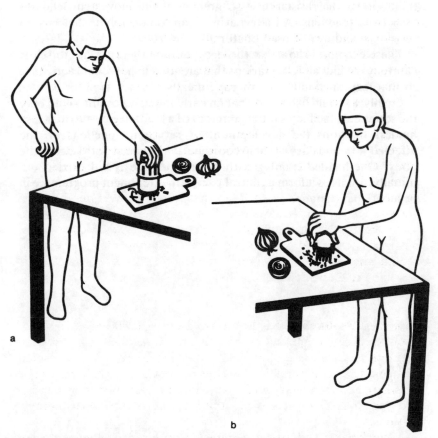

Figures 70a and 70b *(a) Associated reactions during household activities when the affected arm is not incorporated. (b) Using both hands for household activities.*

The adaptation of the workplace of a hemiplegic patient should be such that asymmetrical posture and associated reactions are avoided, if he carries out his professional activities one-handed — for example, when using a typewriter. Symmetrical posture and correct arm positioning are important for all one-handed activities in an office.

Training for one-handed household activities by using various adaptations have to be considered in occupational therapy. During activities the affected side should always be incorporated or at least correctly positioned.

Example. Figure 70a shows the cutting up of onions one-handed using a vegetable chopper. Through the abrupt pushing movements and the tight spring, the resistance is so great that the movement leads to associated reactions. An alternative is an 'onion roller' that has no resistance and can be used bilaterally (Fig 70b).

These examples show that the occupational therapist has to select carefully the aids and adaptations that are used in household activities, so that lost function can be therapeutically compensated for.

Finally, I should like to say that an early intensive training with only the sound side facilitates the asymmetry of a hemiplegic patient. It also hinders or stops the development of returning functions on the affected side, and does not help coordination between both sides of the body. One-handed training with the sound side is not carried out initially, nor does it form a central part of the treatment programme in occupational therapy.

IX Treatment Media

A. Criteria for treatment media
B. Furniture
C. Suitable techniques and activities
D. Remedial games

In chapters V, VI, and VII different media used in treatment and their practical applications were mentioned. A detailed description may be necessary, so in this chapter the most important aspects of the purchase and manufacture of these are considered.

Several different treatment materials are commercially available and only a selection of these are described. The different materials that are necessary and that can be accommodated in the occupational therapy department depends on the size of the department and the kind of clients (besides hemiplegic patients) who are treated there.

A. Criteria for Treatment Media

(1) Stable
(2) Adjustable
(3) Variable
(4) Stimulating

(1) Stable

When purchasing as well as when making treatment media one should ensure that they are stable, strong and secure. They have to be able to withstand constant use. Tables and chairs have to be absolutely secure and angled table-tops should not be allowed to collapse. Equipment made from card should be quite strong and covered with matt transparent plastic in order to avoid reflection.

(2) Adjustable

If a piece of equipment is adjustable and versatile a variety of patients may be treated with it, even though height, disability and the aims of the individual patient may be different. Tables with fixed heights and drawers that obstruct access are not suitable. A vertical sanding board that cannot be adjusted is suitable for only a few patients. Materials and equipment used in techniques and other activities should be adapted and adjusted in such a way that the therapist can achieve an up or down grading in the degree of difficulty.

Examples
Block-printing with interchangeable handles.
Board game with holes so that large, medium or small pieces can be inserted.
Treatment media that have various application possibilities can be used to train perceptual functions as well as motor function.

Example
Practising large arm movements with an open hand may also facilitate spatial perception and constructional ability (Figs 35a, 35b, 35c).
Appropriate planning and execution of different work sequences may be practised bilaterally as well as unilaterally, as shown in Figs 41, 57, and 74. An upgrading is achieved by using nine instead of three pieces.

(3) Variable

A variety of treatment media should be used: only by practising functions with different materials is treatment success made possible.

Example
Gross grip function is practised not only with a small rubber ball but also with fabric, wool, leather and tennis balls, as well as with dice, cylinders, tube and rod-shaped objects. Through this the patient gains experience with hard, soft, thick, thin, short, long, square, round, heavy and light objects.

(4) Stimulating

These media should encourage the patient to use his extremities appropriately.

Example

If one side of the body has been neglected, the aim of treatment should be the spontaneous use of both hands — for example, pottery, weaving, making collages. The anticipation of an end-product will give an incentive for using the hands correctly.

B. Furniture

 (1) Cupboards
 (2) Tables
 (3) Blackboard
 (4) Chairs
 (5) Stools
 (6) Stools on castors
 (7) Footstools
 (8) Benches
 (9) Sanding board
(10) Work benches
(11) Hooks on the wall

The requirements for ADL training areas, a light and heavy workshop, storage facilities as well as office space, vary according to the type of hospital. Good lighting, sufficient electrical outlets, running hot and cold water and a sewing machine are all basic requirements and are not mentioned in detail in this chapter.

(1) Cupboards

If two treatment rooms are adjacent, the separating wall could have a built-in cupboard that is accessible from both rooms. The contents, therefore, do not have to be duplicated. Sliding or folding doors are particularly suitable for a small department.

(2) Tables

For individual treatment the size of a table should ideally be about 120 cm × 80 cm. If two or four tables of the same size are purchased they could be put together during group activities. Raised edges on tables should be avoided because they are a danger to the affected arm, particularly when sensory deficits exist. The tables should be accessible

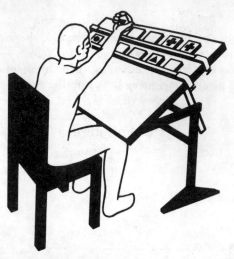

Figure 71. *Hydraulic table with angled top; wooden slats are fixed with clamps and the patient is turning 'Memory' blocks.*

for wheelchair users, and should not have built-in drawers or other hindering accessories underneath. The height and surface should also be adjustable, the latter vertically (see Figs 28; 45a; 45b; 47; 56). To prevent material sliding down from a vertical surface, a non-slip mat may be used. Game boards, table looms and other equipment can be rested on slats, clamped to the table as shown in Fig 71. Magnetic table surfaces are also available.

(3) Blackboard

A large blackboard can be used for painting as well as writing. It should not be fixed to the wall, so that it can be used horizontally, vertically and at any angle as well as when sitting or standing.

An alternative is a laminated surface from which chalk, pencil or water colour drawings may easily be erased. This type of surface is used in preference to large pieces of paper during bilateral or unilateral pre-writing movements. Paper tears easily if movements are not fluent and coordinated.

(4) Chairs

The chairs used in occupational therapy should be solid and should have a straight horizontal seat. Other types of seats are unsuitable. A

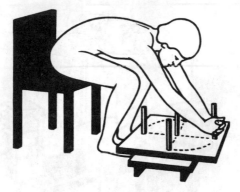

Figure 72. *Remedial game positioned on a foot stool.*

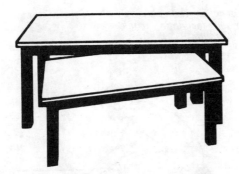

Figure 73. *Two different-sized benches; the small one fits under the larger one.*

mixture of chairs with backrests and armrests, as well as chairs without armrests are used.

(5) Stools

Stools, too, have to be absolutely solid and safe and should be of normal chair height. They are used when practising sitting balance, and as a work surface during some activities (see Figs 7; 13; 35b; 35c; 44).

(6) Stools on Castors

For safety reasons these have five wheels and are used more by the therapist than the patients. They make it easier for the therapist to facilitate large arm movements.

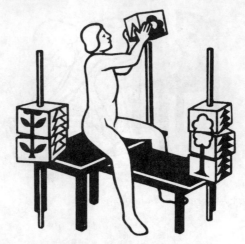

Figure 74. *Use of benches while playing with a large puzzle bimanually facilitating trunk, shoulder and head rotation.*

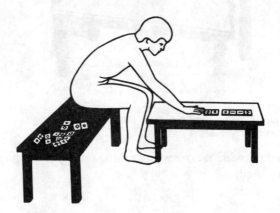

Figure 75. *Playing dominoes.*

(7) Footstools

These should be between 5 cm and 35 cm high. They can be used if the patient's feet do not reach the ground and also as a work surface. As the activity is placed gradually lower and lower the patient practises coming forwards and through this he eventually reaches his feet or the ground (Figs 43; 59; 72).

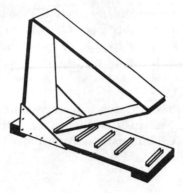

Figure 76. *Sanding board construction.*

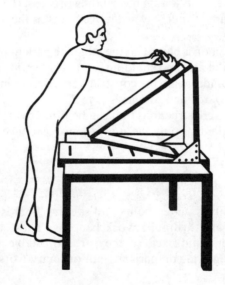

Figure 77. *Positioned on the table for upward movements of the arm while standing.*

(8) Benches

Two benches of different heights are useful pieces of equipment, one measuring 100 cm × 35 cm × 45 cm high, the other 80 cm × 35 cm × 35 cm high. The small one can be put under the large one, which is useful in small departments (Fig 73).

These benches are particularly suitable when the patient is afraid of falling, or during weightbearing activities (Figs 11b; 59). If the patient needs to practise trunk rotation he can sit astride the benches, which eliminates compensatory movements. This is indicated, however, only if the hip does not show abnormal movements like abduction and external rotation (Fig 74).

The lower bench is used with smaller patients as it gives them more security than a higher chair and footstool. This bench also offers a larger work surface during extension movements of the arm (Fig 75).

(9) Sanding Board

An adjustable sanding board is necessary in all occupational therapy departments. The grading should be adjustable for upward as well as downward movements during the sanding process. If it is placed on the floor it can be used for downward movements of the arm while sitting (Figs 76; 36).

If the construction is placed on the table the patient practises upward movements of the arm and standing safety is guaranteed by fixing two pieces of wood underneath the construction, eliminating the possibility of sliding backwards and forwards (Fig 77).

There are also constructions that can be fitted to the wall. Their use, however, is limited, as only the upward movement of the arm can be practised.

(10) Work Benches

Not only are tables, table looms and sanding boards available commercially, but also hydraulic work benches. These are suitable for wheelchair users, and because they are adjustable in height, have certain advantages in comparison with ordinary work benches.

(11) Hooks on the Wall

These should be placed at different heights and are useful for hanging game boards on. The patient practises bilateral or unilateral arm movements while standing.

C. Suitable Techniques and Activities

(1) Painting
(2) Batik
(3) Block-printing
(4) Weaving
(5) Sanding
(6) Woodwork

If craft or other creative activities are used during the treatment of a hemiplegic patient, the therapist has to adapt or simplify the process so that other perceptual functions as well as movements are facilitated.

(1) Painting

Painting may be used at each stage of recovery to practise the various appropriate movement sequences. (It may also have been a hobby of the patient.) If the patient is not interested in painting a picture he can practise the movements by erasing lines and figures from a blackboard, or drawing with a template (Fig 40). In order to work bilaterally the chalk, pen or brush is held with clasped hands (an adaptation to the handle is sometimes necessary). During the later stages painting can also be used as pre-writing practice. If large arm movements are one of the treatment aims, painting on a blackboard or on large sheets of paper, paper batik and the painting of finished products are all suitable to achieve this. If a patient is hesitant because of the empty white sheet of paper he can be asked to paint over a newspaper. Drawing with a ruler or template is mainly used to facilitate the coordination of both hands during bimanual activities.

(2) Batik

The technique of batik on paper, as well as on fabric, offers a variety of movements in functional training. The application of wax may be carried out either bilaterally or unilaterally.

Examples
Wax can be applied to some papers by rubbing a candle over them; more porous ones need melted wax brushed onto them.
One can also let wax from a burning candle drip onto the paper.
Heated wax can be bilaterally applied by holding brushes, cardboard pieces or adapted pastry cutters between clasped hands.

For pre-writing movements a Tjanting may also be used.

If a large piece of paper is used one not only improves the movements of the arm and hand but facilitates sitting balance and the compensation of hemianopia at the same time.

When using tie-dying in the later stages the coordination of both hands is practised.

(3) Block-printing

Blocks are made from lino or cork and ready-made rubber stamps are used for printing on fabric or paper (see also Figs 29; 38a; 38b; 38c; 44). If all blocks and handles have velcro attached they will be interchangeable. Block-printing facilitates motor as well as proprioceptive functions. Through the use of templates patients with limited coordination may also achieve success.

(4) Weaving

This technique is used only when certain arm and hand functions are present. Working at a rug loom or at a differently positioned table loom (vertical, at an angle) the patient achieves good shoulder mobilisation. Figure 47 shows the suitable positioning of the table loom in order to eliminate the undesirable shoulder retraction and elbow flexion. The coordination of both hands is facilitated during 'round weaving' with sisal cord shown in Fig 66. If fine-finger movements need to be practised, finger weaving may be used.

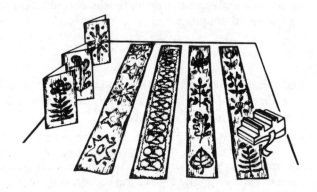

Figure 78. Cards made with the 'colouring technique' using an adapted colouring block.

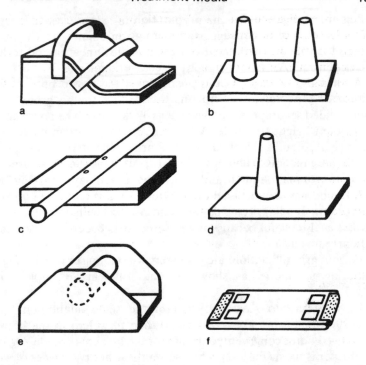

Figures 79a, 79b, 79c, 79d, 79e, 79f and 79g. (a)
Ramp-like block with straps. (b) Vertical cones
for bimanual sanding and colouring.
(c) Horizontal handles for bimanual activities.
(d) Single cone for unilateral and bilateral
activities. (e) Single horizongal handle.
(f) Sanding board, size 11cm × 22cm suitable for
all adapted blocks. (g) Colouring block, size
11cm × 22cm with fixed crayons.

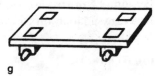

g

(5) Sanding

Most occupational therapy departments have some kind of adapted
sanding construction. Depending on the disability of the patient,
boards are sanded sitting or standing, downwards (Fig 36) or upwards
(Fig 77), unilaterally or bilaterally using various adapted sanding
blocks. The objects that are sanded may also be varied. Frequently
patients, particularly women, do not like this type of activity. Even so,
these movements are a fixed part of treatment in some departments,

and as they are useful for the preparation of arm functions in other activities some different suggestions are given below.

Dried leaves, pillow lace or designs like flowers are fixed to long pieces of wood. A strip of paper is placed over them and fixed at either end. Then the sanding block is pushed over the paper, but this time instead of sandpaper two crayons are fixed into the groove with double-sided sellotape, as shown in Figs 37 and 79g. The board can be fixed at any height and angle. After frequent to and fro movements of this type of colouring block, the designs are visible on paper (similar to the process of brass rubbing). The strip of paper may be used for decoration or may be cut up and used to make birthday cards (Fig 78).

These designs can be used quite often and this technique makes a change from sanding. To achieve an end-product within one treatment session is also useful because it can sometimes cheer up a depressed patient.

Various grip adaptations are necessary for sanding or when using the colouring technique, as shown in the following examples (Figs 79a–79e).

In order not to have two sets of the same adaptations (Figs 79a–79e), one can make one set and then fix velcro to the bottom. Then two boards congruent to the size of the blocks are made. On one, sandpaper is fixed (Fig 79f), whereas on the other two pieces of wood with a groove in the middle of each one are made to hold the crayons (Fig 79g). Both these boards have the other half of the velcro attached. Now any adaptation can be used with either of the two boards.

(6) Woodwork

This is particularly suitable in the later stages of treatment for facilitating normal arm and hand functions, as well as coordination between both hands.

A hydraulic work bench makes it easy to adapt the work environment to each individual patient. It is important to remember that during activities like sawing, planing, rasping, filing or sanding, the extension movements get more resistance and the flexion movements less. Most of the tools have to be adapted for bilateral use. A second handle is put on a saw, rasp and file.

D. Remedial Games

When using remedial games as treatment media, there are other additional criteria to take into consideration apart from the ones mentioned under section A.

When buying or making remedial games good quality material should be used. If the media are pleasant and stimulating then they are useful. It is also important to use materials that stimulate sensation — for example, covering pieces of a game with different fabrics, making numbers with pimply rubber (Fig 25).

If a game is enlarged the therapist must decide on the most suitable size for the pieces without making them too big. It is also important to remember that if a patient knows the original version or has a hemianopia it may be difficult for him to adapt.

To make a remedial game variable two factors have to be taken into consideration. Firstly, the game should offer the opportunity of training appropriate motor functions in the various stages of recovery. This may be achieved through the different shapes and sizes of the pieces. Secondly, the therapist should not see the training of motor functions in isolation and disregard other perceptual dysfunctions. Remedial games should be made simpler and easier — for example, through changing the rules.

It should be remembered that the remedial game is adapted for adults. Even if other brain functions are affected the games should not be childish.

When choosing a game the time to complete it should be considered. The remedial game should be only part of a treatment session so that other activities may be incorporated. Games like chess are unsuitable.

Some of the various games suitable in the treatment of an adult hemiplegic patient are described below.

(1) Board games
(2) Number-pushing game
(3) 'Memory'
(4) Dominoes
(5) Span games
(6) Puzzles
(7) Skittles
(8) Dice games

(1) Board Games

Of the different board games the therapist chooses the ones that are best known, most widely used and which need a variety of movement sequences. Some are useful as they are, others need to be adapted. In the treatment stages 1–4 (chapter V) the original version may be used during the functional training.

Particularly useful is 'Othello'. During the weightbearing activities in the early stages of treatment, whether sitting or standing, forwards or sideways, the treatment aim is not the static supporting of the arm but the active weight transference onto the affected arm. If 'Othello' is played in stage 1 of recovery with the sound hand, the board is placed next to the weightbearing affected arm. All the pieces, however, are as far away from that point as possible. As each move in the game needs a new piece the desired weight transfer with active movement of the patient's body is achieved, facilitating sitting or standing balance at the same time. If the adapted versions of this game (bigger and smaller) are used during stage 4, it is played with the affected hand. As the rules demand that pieces should be added and reversed, this game requires frequent repetition of movement sequences.

A square board measuring 55 cm × 55 cm × 4 cm may be used in the adaptation of the various games. Both sides of the board can have a game mapped out. The holes should have a diameter of 2.5 cm and should be deep enough to prevent the pieces from falling out if the game is used vertically.

Examples. On one side could be a game of solitaire (Figs 43; 45; 51; 63). This game is favourable for functional training in occupational therapy, because it requires frequent repetition of movement sequences. On the other side could be 'Nine-Men's Morris' (Fig 28).

Another board could have 'Othello' (64 holes; 8 cm × 8 cm rows) on one side with Draughts on the other (Fig 26).

With these adapted board games a variety of pieces can be used. All the pieces can be put into the holes or placed on the board. With such a variety the therapist may undertake sensory-motor training using bilateral movements and practise gross motor prehension as well as fine skilled manipulations.

(a) Rods, about 14 cm long, diameter 2.5 cm. These are made out of broom handles, painted in two different colours and are

bilaterally picked up with clasped hands (Figs 26; 27; 28). Later
on they are also used to practise grip functions.

(b) Sixty-four pieces of dowelling are painted half in one colour,
half in another. These are the 'Othello' pieces and can only be
used unilaterally.

(c) In order to combine motor with sensory training the rods are
covered with different materials (Fig 51).

(d) Wooden or rubber balls with a diameter of about 6 cm placed
onto the holes in the board, are used for training early grip
functions. If the patient has insufficient control over his movements, however, they may roll away.

(e) Balls made out of different fabrics and filled with different
materials varying in weight and consistency, are used during the
training of deep as well as superficial sensation.

(f) With severe sensory deficits the therapist chooses balls with
gross differences (Fig 63).

(g) Round balls with a diameter of 6 cm attached to a piece of
dowelling, with a diameter of 2.5 cm are suitable for early grip
functions (Figs 43; 45).

(h) The hammer top game piece (top rod diameter of about 4 cm) is
a variation of the ball grip, practising early grip and grip-release
functions.

(i) A rod with a magnet attached (see section on Memory and
Puzzles) gives another opportunity to play a game bilaterally
with clasped hands. This time the pieces consist of round discs
with a drawing pin attached to them. These pieces are put into
the holes with the help of the magnet.

(j) In the late stages of recovery, shorter pieces are used which
stick out of the hole by only 1 cm or 2 cm. If an eyelet is inserted
into the pieces, fine skilled motor functions may be practised in
combination with large arm movements.

By using such adapted remedial games as treatment media, the
therapist can achieve the different treatment aims of a hemiplegic
patient. The board may be placed low (Figs 43; 72), high (Fig 26),
horizontal (Fig 27), at an angle (Figs 28; 45a; 45b) or vertical (Fig 26).
The pieces of the games are placed in such a way that the patient has to
change from one reflex inhibiting position to the next, thereby facilitating normal movement sequences as well as trunk rotation (Figs 12; 27;
45).

(2) Number-Pushing Game

This type of game is commercially available as a 'pocket game': 15 or 23 numbers should be put into sequence through pushing them vertically or horizontally.

As a treatment medium the game is enlarged. A smooth board (48 cm × 72 cm) with a low lip around it is constructed. The edges of the 23 squares (12 cm × 12 cm) are rounded and the underside must be very smooth to ensure easy movements. The figures are painted on or are cut out of pimply rubber and then glued on.

The use of this game with motor deficits during the different stages of recovery of hemiplegia, are as follows.

(a) If the rectangle frame is placed widthways in front of the patient, the therapist achieves abduction of the arm, weight transfer from one side to the other, facilitation of sitting balance and, if applicable, compensation for a hemianopia.

(b) If the treatment aims are arm extension and shoulder protraction, and perhaps leaning forwards, the frame is placed lengthwise in front of the patient.

(c) The number squares are pushed bilaterally with clasped hands either at table height or lower (Fig 25).

(d) Unilateral pushing with the affected hand is at first possible only with the help of the therapist. Later, less and less help is given (Figs 35a; 35b; 35c). Through pushing with the heel of the hand, extension of wrist and fingers is achieved.

(e) To encourage coordination between both hands at a later stage, the frame is placed at an angle. The squares will now tend to fall down and will have to be kept in place with one hand while the other hand pushes.

(f) If the game is played one-handed while still at an angle, extension and abduction as well as adduction of the fingers and thumb are practised. This is possible only at a very late stage.

Into this frame a number of other games may be inserted to make treatment more variable or to train perceptual functions.

(a) To make it easier for the patient only 12 numbers in two rows, or 15 numbers on 16 squares are used. The unused space is filled with neutral squares. If one allows two empty squares the process of sequencing is also made easier.

(b) Squares with shapes or colours may be sorted by pushing (Fig 35b).

(c) A picture or a clockface may be inserted.

(d) If lines are painted on the squares, geometric shapes may be built (Fig 35c). As this is a task that falls into the area of two-dimensional construction ability, it might be too difficult for the patient.

(e) Equally demanding is the construction of a colour sequence.

(f) If letters are painted on the squares words can be constructed horizontally as well as vertically in the form of a simple crossword puzzle.

(g) If two of the four rows are made neutral through empty squares, the other 16 squares may be used to solve 'problems'.

No Contact. Four different colours are used to paint 16 squares, four squares to each colour. These squares should be placed so that two of the same colour are not next to each other. Here vertical and horizontal as well as diagonal direction has to be considered.

Small Magical Square. The coloured squares are given a certain number value — for example, red = 1; green = 2; yellow = 3; and blue = 4. During insertion of the colour–number–symbols the patient is asked to ensure that the sum of the four vertical, the four horizontal and the two diagonal rows, as well as the sum of the four small squares, is always ten.

Magical Square. The pieces 1–15 have to be placed onto 16 spaces so that the sum of the four vertical, four horizontal and the two diagonal number rows, as well as the sum of the four small squares, is always 30.

(h) Fifty-four wooden blocks with velcro attached can be placed into this frame as described in the 'Memory' section. With their measurements (8cm × 8cm) they are a useful size for practising gross motor prehension. If a poster (72 cm × 48 cm) is glued on a piece of cardboard and then cut up into 54 square pieces that have the other half of the velcro attached, they can be put onto the wooden blocks, and one has a large puzzle that fits into the frame.

This variety of pushing games offers several possible ways of treating the individual. Using these media the therapist can achieve different treatment aims at the same time — for example, both the facilitation of motor function and the training of perceptual functions — in the various stages of recovery.

(3) 'Memory'

This is a placing game with pairs of cards that can be varied — for example, pictures, shapes, numbers, words and also a combination of, say, pictures and words. It demands the ability to remember and concentrate as well as the spatial orientation of the patient.

As a preparation, the matching of two of the same cards can be practised in combination with functional movements of the arm — for example, during the early stage bilateral matching with clasped hands or with abducted-extended fingers (Fig 31) may be practised. As movement functions of the arm and hand improve, unilateral matching can take place, as in Fig 34, until this is also possible with grip functions.

In order to play the game 'Memory' in the early stage, a paperclip is fastened to each card. A magnet is attached to a piece of dowelling (15 cm long) which is held between clasped hands. The magnet is not placed straight onto the paperclip but diagonally — almost horizontally. Through this the card is lifted and then turned over (Fig 80).

The movement sequence is not very clear in the figure, and is also difficult for some patients. Nevertheless, through the positioning of hands and the curiosity to see the card, the therapist can facilitate head position, the level of the shoulder and the rotation of the arm.

Before practising the fine motor skills that are needed for turning the cards over in the later stage of recovery, the game may be adapted so that pronation and supination with gross prehension are practised.

The 'Memory' cards can be mounted onto wooden dice (16 cm square) with glue or with velcro. This facilitates grip function. If supination is limited, two movements can be made at 90°. As an alternative, wooden blocks 8 cm × 8 cm square and 1–2 cm, sometimes 4 cm high can be made. One surface has the loops of the velcro attached. The 'Memory' cards are 8 cm × 8 cm square and have the hooks of the velcro attached. Different cards or puzzle pieces may be attached to the wooden block.

This game can be played at different heights — for example, on a low bench, at table height (Fig 46) or on a table surface placed at an angle (Fig 71).

(4) Dominoes

The original number version can be varied by using pictures, shapes, colours or other complementing objects. Dominoes in their original

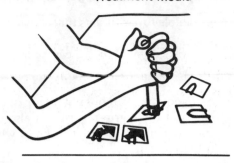

Figure 80. *Turning 'Memory' cards with a magnet attached to a wooden rod.*

size of about 2 cm × 4 cm or 4 cm × 8 cm are suitable for pushing with clasped hands or abducted fingers.

To practise pushing extension movements of the arm, or the grip functions of the hand during unilateral use of the affected upper extremity, the therapist can enlarge them.

(a) Forty-five pieces made of wood (size 8 cm × 16 cm × 1.5 cm) are painted with nine different shapes in nine different colours. On the other side numbers from one to nine with dots are indicated in the same nine colours in regular distribution.

Variation. Six different shapes and the numbers 1–6 are indicated with dots on only 21 pieces. If all doubles are now removed one is left with 15 pieces. This makes the game easier for the patient.

(b) The wooden blocks described in the 'Memory' section may also be used for domino cards — for example, a circle. Each half of it is on a different domino card and through the correct choice the full circle is shown.

Unilateral training is carried out in the first place on a low bench (Fig 75). In order to select the correct domino with the sound hand, the affected one is used in the weightbearing position, as shown in Fig 11b. This combination of pushing and weightbearing may also be used while standing at a work bench or at a long high table.

The domino pieces described under (a) and (b) are again useful for grip function when practised on a bench or at table height. One also selects movement sequences as shown in Figs 45a and 45b. They can also be played at an angled table top with slats that are clamped on the table as in Fig 71.

Apart from the various ways domino pieces can be made, methods of playing the game may also be varied.

The domino pieces are not matched but put on top of each other. This demands not only controlled grip-release but also concentration and memory from the patient, in order to know which of the halves he has to join the piece to.

With the same piece he can match according to shape (disregarding colour) or number (disregarding colour) and another time according to colour (disregarding shape and number). Different uses of the same game enable the therapist to train motor function in a varied way. It also demands adaptability from the patient because he has to think about the system that is in use at any one time.

Matching is not done with the same number, but so that the sum of both adjoining halves is always 10.

The understanding of symbols is usually carried out with brain-injured patients in paper pencil exercises. This can, however, be combined with the training of motor functions — for example, the shape dominoes are given number symbols (circle = 1; square = 2; cross = 3 and so on), then the patient can be asked to match two domino halves that add up to 10.

A constant readjustment is demanded from the patient if shape–symbol–number has to be matched alternately with numbers on normal pieces, so that the sum is always 10.

These variations of dominoes are useful treatment media that are adjustable to any stage of recovery during the rehabilitation of an adult hemiplegic patient.

(5) Span Games

This game consists of three rods and four to six discs of different sizes. All the discs are sorted, according to size, onto one of the rods and are then transferred onto the third rod without a larger one being placed over a smaller one.

Even with good planning this rule demands a constant change of the discs from one rod to another. By using this game the patient achieves constant repetition of the necessary movement functions.

Large bilateral arm movements with slight external rotation and supination are gained if the game is enlarged. With a diameter of

10–40 cm and a height of 10 cm, these discs have to be made out of very light wood, and be hollow or made out of polystyrene. To fix the pieces of dowel, metal tubes are welded onto clamps, either vertically or at an angle. A screw inserted into the metal rod keeps the dowel at the desired height. Depending on the motor functions that need practising, these rods are offered to the patient either vertically or at an angle.

A variation of this game may be played sitting on a bench (Fig 74), making trunk rotation necessary. If these three rods are clamped to a table or a work bench, the patient practises weight transfers standing or even side stepping (Fig 41).

During the final stages a small version with thin discs for skilled span grip training may be chosen (Fig 54). If these need to be combined with large arm movements, the three rods are placed quite far apart.

(6) Puzzles

These come in many different varieties, some with straight, others with round, cutouts. Their degree of difficulty depends on the size and contrast of foreground and background, as well as on the number of pieces. Some Chinese geometric puzzles and of mosaic-making belong in this category.

When using puzzles, the therapist has to take the ability of form and space perception of the patient into consideration. During the early stages of treatment a puzzle can be constructed with the sound hand, while weightbearing occurs through the affected arm (see also Figs 11a; 11b; 53). The pieces of a large wooden puzzle are fitted with a drawing pin and the patient can assemble them with the help of a magnet. In the later stages, when bilateral arm movements are possible, enlarged rods may be used (see previous section) to assemble pictures vertically (Fig 74).

Before grip functions are good enough to manipulate small puzzle pieces, one can practise gross prehension with 8 cm × 8 cm wooden blocks covered with pictures. These can be put into the frame that was used for the number-pushing game.

(7) Skittles

Hemiplegic patients with other perceptual deficits are often depressed, because they cannot achieve certain things. The combined treatment of motor as well as perceptual dysfunction is often too demanding and they have to be practised separately. Playing skittles is a useful motor function training for such patients.

With the patient seated on a chair, it can be played bilaterally or unilaterally at a large table or on the floor. The weight transfer forwards (Fig 72) facilitates sitting balance and prepares the patient for activities of daily living, as well as for standing up.

Rods or large domino pieces may be used instead of skittles. If these are placed in a large semicircle around the patient, various arm movement combinations are facilitated as well as compensation training for an existing hemianopia.

In the early stages, the ball is grasped bilaterally high above the head. The patient can hold it between the thumb and index finger of his sound hand. The ball is then put between both feet and pushed forwards. The next one is also picked up high in order to have a contrasting movement. Before grip functions are possible, one can roll the ball unilaterally with the back of the hand, with the arm hanging down (Fig 33). Large light balls made from polystyrene or cork may be used. Trunk rotation is facilitated if the arms swing from the side.

(8) Dice Games

Dice are partly used in combination with board as well as card games. There are also pure dice games and several available books illustrate these. (Most use dice with the numbers 1–6, but there are other ones.) Some pure dice games require mathematical thinking on the patient's part and this is often incorporated into the treatment plan in occupational therapy. Figure 30 shows how the patient can use the dice in a bilateral manner. With clasped hands the dice is held between index finger and thumb of the sound hand resulting in supination of the affected arm.

A large foam dice (about 20 cm square) is held between clasped hands (like a large cardboard box or a large ball) and then thrown on the floor. To practise early grip and grip-release, larger than normal dice are used (about 4–5 cm square). A plate covered with a piece of leather is useful for throwing the dice onto.

In the later stage, a dice-shaker is useful for practising pronation and supination, as well as the coordination of both hands.

Final Note

The treatment media described in this book, particularly in the last chapter, are only a selection of those used in the treatment of an adult hemiplegic patient in occupational therapy.

Under no circumstances should the therapist make the mistake of developing these into rigid exercises. The use of these media should be looked upon as part of a mosaic. In order to complete it the therapist has to establish a treatment plan that is tailored to the individual's needs, incorporating sensory-motor training for functional activities, as well as taking psychological effects into consideration. There are, of course, other media that are useful in the treatment of adult hemiplegia that are not mentioned here. Any suggestions and opinions of colleagues would be of great interest to me.

Index